The Social Nature of Antibiotic Overprescription in China

Offering a rarely seen glimpse into the realities of one of the biggest global public health crises in modern time, Wang's book focuses on doctor–patient interactions in China to demonstrate the potential effects of health communication, doctor–patient relationship, and a matrix of social factors on overprescription of antibiotics.

Based on a community-based survey, the book describes empirical findings regarding the high prevalence of non-prescribed antibiotics use for common colds among children in China. It covers the potential effects of overprescription on caregivers' attitudes and how physicians make prescribing decisions in medical consultations. Drawing from evidence in medical interaction data, readers are introduced to further empirical findings regarding the communicative behaviors that patient caregivers use to pressure for antibiotic prescriptions in real medical consultations. Following this, Wang reports findings regarding the communicative behaviors that physicians use to make treatment recommendations and caregivers use to launch treatment negotiations, leading to a discussion of the effect of the doctor–patient relationship on antibiotic overprescription. The book culminates in practice recommendations and provides teaching scenarios in which physicians successfully engage the caregivers into conversations to shape their expectations for antibiotic prescriptions in medical consultations.

An important resource for scholars and students in health communication, linguistics, medical humanities, and medical sociology. Practitioners who are interested in understanding and improving clinical practices as well as policymakers aiming to combat antibiotic resistance will also find this book useful.

Nan Christine Wang is an Associate Professor in the School of Public Administration at Hunan University, China.

Routledge Studies in Language, Health and Culture

Series Editor: Olga Zayts

University of Hong Kong, Hong Kong

This series has several distinctive features. First, it investigates health communication through linguistic lenses. The contributions introduce the readers to a range of linguistic approaches, including, but not limited to (critical) discourse analysis, sociolinguistics, multimodal analysis, corpus analysis, conversation analysis. Each volume draws on authentic empirical data from a range of healthcare contexts, going beyond the traditional doctor–patient encounters and expanding the focus of inquiry.

Second, the series focuses specifically on contexts outside of the mainstream English-dominant healthcare contexts, encouraging proposals from contributors working on healthcare communication in Asia-Pacific, South America and continental Europe.

Third, some contributions focus on multicultural and multilingual healthcare encounters, thus making the series of relevance to a broad readership around the world.

The series encourages contributions that, in addition to advancing the linguistic field, also stress relevance to professional practice.

Doctor–patient Communication in Chinese and Western Medicine
Ying Jin

The Role of Language in Eastern and Western Health Communication
Jack Pun

Language, Health and Culture
Problematizing the Centers and Peripheries of Healthcare Communication Research
Olga Zayts-Spence and Susan M. Bridges

The Social Nature of Antibiotic Overprescription in China
Medical Conversations, Doctor–Patient Relationships, and Decision-Making
Nan Christine Wang

For more details on the series, please visit: https://www.routledge.com/Routledge-Studies-in-Language-Health-and-Culture/book-series/RSLHC

The Social Nature of Antibiotic Overprescription in China

Medical Conversations, Doctor–Patient Relationships, and Decision-Making

Nan Christine Wang

Routledge
Taylor & Francis Group

LONDON AND NEW YORK

First published 2024
by Routledge
4 Park Square, Milton Park, Abingdon, Oxon OX14 4RN

and by Routledge
605 Third Avenue, New York, NY 10158

Routledge is an imprint of the Taylor & Francis Group, an informa business

© 2024 Nan Christine Wang

British Library Cataloguing-in-Publication Data
A catalogue record for this book is available from the British Library

ISBN: 978-1-032-15324-7 (hbk)
ISBN: 978-1-032-15325-4 (pbk)
ISBN: 978-1-003-24362-5 (ebk)

DOI: 10.4324/9781003243625

Typeset in Times New Roman
by Apex CoVantage, LLC

Contents

Acknowledgment

This is a long overdue acknowledgment.

First and foremost, I would like to express my gratitude to my PhD advisors, John Heritage and Tanya Stivers, who co-chaired my dissertation research in UCLA's sociology department. The contents of this book largely stem from my dissertation research. This book is a product of their inspiration and would not exist without their guidance and support.

The numerous discussions I had with John over the years have shaped my understanding of the problem addressed in this book and helped me discover the excitement and energy inherent in conducting social science research. Over the years, John encouraged me to approach my research from various angles, breaking the boundaries between disciplines. He demonstrated how conversation analysis and sociology can contribute to understanding the problem and how to view it through the lens of history, organization, and culture. He taught me to untangle the complexities of our social world by leveraging the diversity of interdisciplinary perspectives and methodologies, maintaining flexibility to shift between micro and macro levels, between past and future. John's sincere interest and curiosity in our social world, especially its complexity, is what I observed in his work and guidance. This is what I find most enjoyable in my own research and what I hope to share with my students in my career.

Tanya's research on antibiotic prescribing decision-making is the most important source of inspiration and starting point for my dissertation and this book. Her grounded analysis demonstrated how micro-level evidence can be systematically organized to address macro-level issues. This sheds light not only on antibiotic prescribing decision-making in clinical settings but also on how members of society coordinate to achieve their goals and manage relationships. It shows how various dilemmas and conflicts that pervade our social life are formed in our everyday interactions and how they can be dealt with through a thorough understanding of them. Through discussions, data sessions, and lectures, Tanya has consistently encouraged me to question my assumptions through rigorous analysis and pushed me to think further. Her genuine care and kindness have helped me overcome difficulties in my career and personal growth, even after completing my graduate studies.

I would also like to thank Donald Morisky, Stefan Timmermans, and Hongyin Tao, my dissertation committee members. Each of them came from a different disciplinary background and provided enormous help and guidance throughout my dissertation research process. With his mentorship, Donald familiarized me with the perspective that public health researchers often adopt while encouraging me to explore the antibiotic overprescription problem from a social and interactional approach. Through his teaching, Stefan introduced me to the core theoretical issues that medical sociologists seek to address as well as a wide range of analytical tools that they can use in research practice. During his seminars and our discussions, Hongyin introduced me to important theories and concepts related to Chinese linguistics, which were essential components of the analytical approach that I took to answer my research questions.

I would also like to extend my thanks to the participants of this study, including the doctors and patient caregivers, for supporting this research and agreeing to have their medical consultations recorded and analyzed. I am particularly grateful for the kind assistance of the doctors in the consultation room, who facilitated this research despite their already heavy workload. Their generous sharing of opinions and knowledge was also essential to the completion of this study.

In addition, I am indebted to Wei Zhang, my MPhil research advisor at City University of Hong Kong, and Kang Kwong Luke at Nanyang Technological University in Singapore, who was the external examiner of my master thesis at that time. They not only sparked my interest in conducting research on conversation analysis but also provided substantial help and support to continue my research on social interaction in medical settings.

I would also like to express my gratitude to Olga Zayts-Spence and Katie Peace for conceptualizing and creating this book series and for their unwavering support and assistance throughout the writing process. The valuable suggestions from many scholars that I received in conferences and seminars and in reviewing processes have also helped me enormously to improve the work.

Lastly, I extend my deepest thanks to my family for their constant love, support, and understanding. In memory of Luna, thank you for your loving companionship.

1 Introduction

Antibiotic overprescription and associated bacterial resistance have been identified by the World Health Organization (WHO) as one of the biggest global public health crises in the world today. China's antibiotic overuse problem is particularly concerning – as the world's largest manufacturer and second largest consumer of antibiotics, prescription rates of antibiotics have been high, and the resistance rates of multiple strains of bacteria have been growing rapidly. With the high frequency of international travel and exchange, the overuse and inappropriate use of antibiotics in China is not only an alarming issue domestically but also a global public health threat.

To explain what contributes to the high prevalence of antibiotic overprescription in China, most existing research has approached the problem from a health economics perspective, concluding that overprescription is a supply-side problem driven by financial incentives for doctors to overprescribe. As a result, policy decisions direct resources toward changing only the supply-side (provider-related) factors, leaving the demand-side (patient-related) factors largely neglected and unattended.

Nonetheless, a large body of research in Western literature has revealed that demand-side factors could significantly affect antibiotic overprescription – patient desires have been recurrently cited by doctors as the most common reason for overprescribing; perceived parental expectations for prescriptions have been found to increase the likelihood of doctors' inappropriate prescriptions significantly. Thus, overprescribing can result from doctors responding to actual or perceived pressure from the patients or caregivers.

Despite the scale and the magnitude of the problem, to date, a thorough understanding of antibiotic overprescription in China is still lacking. Although supply-side factors were important contributors during a particular period in history, they may not be the only driving force and not even the dominant one as time goes on and the healthcare system evolves. In fact, many intervention measures have been taken to address the problem from the supply side, yet these interventions have only seen limited results.

In this study, I expand the theoretical lens by showing how the supply-side and demand-side behaviors are intertwined and how the prescribing decisions are interactively constructed in social encounters. Moreover, I also aim to

DOI: 10.4324/9781003243625-1

connect the micro-level findings of doctor-caregiver behaviors to the macro-level factors relating to the healthcare system's organization, the country's historical transformation, and the shaping of a medical culture saturated with antibiotics.

Antibiotic resistance and antibiotic overprescription

Antibiotic resistance as a global public health crisis

Unlike a pandemic outbreak, the effects of antimicrobial resistance (AMR) accumulate, and its consequences are often overlooked. When AMR occurs, common infections become harder or impossible to treat, resulting in prolonged hospital stays, higher medical costs, and increased mortality (WHO, 2020a, 2020b). The global burden of AMR could be as many as 10 million deaths by 2050, and the cost to the economy might be as high as US $100 trillion (CDC, 2021; Murray et al., 2022; O'Neil, 2015). Moreover, modern health systems that rely heavily on antibiotics could be severely undermined (Laxminarayan et al., 2013a; O'Neil, 2015). Many medical procedures, such as surgery, organ transplants, or cancer chemotherapy, could lose effectiveness, posing a severe threat to modern medicine (Chan, 2011; Horton, 2019).

Antibiotic resistance is an important form of antimicrobial resistance. Although antibiotic resistance occurs naturally, misuse and overuse of antibiotics in humans and animals contribute to the growth of antibiotic resistance and accelerate the process. The problem is further exacerbated by the fact that the pipeline for developing new antibiotics is running dry (Boucher et al., 2009; Shlaes et al., 2013), as the pharmaceutical industry lacks the financial incentives to develop new antibiotics that could cure conditions in weeks rather than years (Brogan & Mossialos, 2013). In countries around the world, many antibiotics are prescribed inappropriately for viral conditions that are self-limiting, such as common colds, viral sore throats, and ear infections (Hicks et al., 2015; Fleming-Dutra et al., 2016; Nowakowska et al., 2019).

Although the problem has been widely recognized and addressed by many high-income countries, it is relatively insufficiently recognized in low- and middle-income countries and regions (Laxminarayan et al., 2013b, 2016). For instance, in France, Sweden, and the United States, successful interventions have been implemented and gratifying progress has been made to reduce resistance rates in the past two decades (Hicks et al., 2015; Kronman et al., 2020; Mölstad et al., 2008; Sabuncu et al., 2009); whereas in countries such as Brazil, China, and India, resistance levels have escalated rapidly during the same period (Laxminarayan et al., 2016; WHO, 2014).

China is at the heart of this crisis. More than 200 types of antibiotics are consumed a year, amounting to approximately 162 million tons (Zhang et al., 2015). The resistance rates of many types of pathogens – methicillin-resistant *staphylococci*, erythromycin-insensitive *S. pneumoniae*, and fluoroquinolone-resistant *E. coli* – are high (CARSS, 2016; Mei & Tong, 2012; Xiao et al., 2008). Inappropriate antibiotic prescribing can be observed across various clinical settings (Wang et al., 2014; Zhao et al., 2021). In primary care outpatient settings, 52.9% of prescriptions contained antibiotics, of which only 39.4% were considered appropriate

(Wang et al., 2014). In the context of acute upper respiratory infections (AURIs), where overprescription is most likely to happen, 63.2% of the antibiotics prescribed were not in line with clinical guidelines (Zhao et al., 2020).

Conflicting theories on China's problem and research gap

The high prevalence of antibiotic overprescription in China is a subject of debate in current literature. Research in Western countries has mostly argued that antibiotic overprescription is a demand-side problem, with patient pressure being the main reason for doctors to prescribe inappropriately (Ong et al., 2007; Scott et al., 2001). However, the Chinese literature largely attributes the problem to the supply side, blaming doctors who overprescribe for financial gain (Currie et al., 2011; Li et al., 2012; Reynolds & McKee, 2009; Yip et al., 2014).

The demand-side theory: the Western and the Chinese cases

Patient influence on antibiotic overprescription has been most extensively examined in Western clinical settings. In addition to studies that use survey instruments or interview methods (Fletcher-Lartey et al., 2016; Kumar et al., 2003; Linder & Singer, 2003; O'Connor et al., 2018; Ong et al., 2007), research that investigates naturally occurring medical interactions in American pediatric settings also presents substantial evidence that perceived parental pressure significantly affects doctors' prescribing behavior (Mangione-Smith et al., 1999, 2001, 2006; Stivers, 2007). Although overt requests from parents for antibiotics were rare, covert forms of pressure can be observed throughout the various stages of medical consultations (Stivers, 2002b, 2002a; Stivers & Timmermans, 2020, 2021). For instance, *candidate diagnosis,* through which caregivers seek confirmation of a bacterial infection diagnosis and indicate the relevance of antibiotic treatment, can be used to advocate for antibiotics (Stivers, 2002b); *resistance to non-antibiotic treatment recommendations*, through which caregivers initiate a negotiation for antibiotic treatment can also be observed as a practice to advocate for antibiotic treatment (Stivers, 2005).

Contrary to the prevailing focus on patients' influence in the Western literature, patients' impact on antibiotic overprescription in China has received much less attention. Few studies investigated patients' impact, and almost all concluded that doctors are the main reason for the problem (Currie et al., 2011; He, 2014). For instance, one study using an experimental design reported that when standard patients displayed knowledge of antibiotics, doctors were less likely to prescribe them inappropriately (Currie et al., 2011). It is only recently that researchers started to find conflicting evidence about patients' influence on antibiotic overprescription (Wang, 2020; Wang & Liu, 2021; Wang et al., 2023).

The supply-side theory: the Western and the Chinese cases

In the Western literature, many studies that focus on naturally occurring medical interaction examine doctors' role in overprescription under the premise that doctor–patient communication can be improved to manage parental expectations for unwarranted antibiotic prescriptions. For instance, in American pediatric settings, *online commentary* is found to be a practice used to prepare patients and caregivers for non-antibiotic treatment recommendations, maximizing the chance for their acceptance (Heritage et al., 2010; Heritage & Stivers, 1999). Relatedly, how doctors deliver non-antibiotic treatment recommendations has been examined regarding their impact on patient and caregiver resistance (Stivers, 2005). Specifically, Stivers (2005) found that a positively framed recommendation (e.g., *I'm gonna give her some cough medicine*) is less likely to engender parent resistance than a negatively framed one (e.g., *She doesn't need any antibiotics*). In British primary care consultations for children, although researchers found evidence that parents actually tend to avoid antibiotics and their communication rarely implies an expectation for antibiotics, the study is similarly rested upon the premise that doctors' prescribing decisions are likely to be influenced by perceived parental expectations for antibiotics (Cabral et al., 2014, 2019).

In sum, while extensive attention has been given to the influence of patients on antibiotic overprescription in Western countries and the influence of perverse incentives on the part of doctors in Chinese clinical settings, our understanding of the antibiotic overprescription problem in China remains incomplete. This incomplete understanding has consequences, as failure to recognize the evolving reasons for the problem will leave it unresolved and render previous efforts to address it futile. This study is thus motivated by these considerations.

Road map of the book

The following chapters are organized as described next.

Chapter 2 focuses on the historical and institutional factors contributing to the problem. I begin by describing a typical medical visit from a patient caregiver's perspective, showing what a patient goes through before and during a medical visit when they have common acute respiratory tract infection symptoms, such as cough and fever. I then briefly describe the Chinese healthcare system's historical evolution and institutional arrangement, aiming to contextualize these medical visits, which I will examine closely in this study. Following this, I point out a matrix of perverse incentives attributable to the antibiotic overprescription problem, encompassing the individual doctor, the hospital, the pharmaceutical industry, and the organization of the healthcare system. The chapter concludes by discussing the spillover effect of these macro-level factors on shaping a medical culture saturated with antibiotic prescriptions.

In the following chapters, I steer our attention to the factors related to the medical encounters where antibiotic prescribing decisions are made and show that antibiotic prescribing decisions are socially influenced by patient caregivers and interactionally negotiated in naturally occurring conversations.

Chapter 3 examines patient caregivers' influence on antibiotic prescribing decisions, even before their interaction with doctors in medical visits. It investigates patient caregivers' pre-visit use of non-prescribed antibiotics for common cold symptoms, caregivers' expectations for antibiotic prescriptions, the prescriptions they receive in the medical visits, and the relationship between these factors. Socioeconomic characteristics of the caregiver and clinical characteristics of the patient's condition that predict higher rates of pre-visit use of non-prescribed antibiotics and expectations for antibiotics are discussed.

Chapter 4 focuses on patient caregivers' influence on prescribing decisions in and through their communicative practices within medical visits. Specifically, I examine four interactional behaviors that they use and that are often understood by doctors as advocating for antibiotic prescriptions. On the qualitative side, I show what these practices are like and how they are understood and responded to by doctors in medical interaction. Moreover, the effects of these communicative practices on prescribing decisions are also examined quantitatively.

Chapter 5 examines doctors' role in antibiotic overprescription by analyzing the content and the action design of their treatment recommendations in medical visits. I start from the theoretical assumption that if the problem is predominantly doctor-driven, one would see doctors recommend antibiotics to their patients vigorously, asserting a high level of authority. I then present findings from conversation analyses of naturally occurring conversations that (1) although doctors do not recommend a significantly large amount of antibiotics, they end up prescribing more and (2) their treatment recommendation actions are more commonly delivered in a way that embodies a relatively low level of medical authority.

Chapter 6 examines the relative effect of the doctors and the caregivers by examining the treatment recommendation-response sequence in prescribing decision-making interaction. A detailed analysis of the sequential unfolding of these sequences shows that (1) patient caregivers are not passive followers of doctors – they actively participate in the prescribing decision-making by resisting doctors' treatment recommendations, initiating negotiation for desirable treatment (mostly antibiotic) and (2) in the face of caregivers' resistance, doctors pursue caregivers' acceptance of their original recommendation (mostly non-antibiotic) in a majority of cases.

Chapter 7 concludes the book by revisiting the research question and summarizing the key findings of each chapter. I then highlight the contribution of these findings by pointing to the gaps that the study fills in the research landscape. Importantly, I show the complementary relationship between the micro-level and macro-level factors rather than pose them as conflicting and mutually independent.

Appendix 1 offers some notes on data and methods used in this study as well as a note on the transcribing symbols that are used in producing the data excerpts shown in the book.

References

Boucher, H. W., Talbot, G. H., Bradley, J. S., Edwards, J. E., Gilbert, D., Rice, L. B., Scheld, M., Spellberg, B., & Bartlett, J. (2009). Bad bugs, no drugs: No ESKAPE! An update from the Infectious Diseases Society of America. *Clinical Infectious Diseases: An Official Publication of the Infectious Diseases Society of America*, *48*(1), 1–12. https://doi.org/10.1086/595011

Brogan, D. M., & Mossialos, E. (2013). Incentives for new antibiotics: The Options Market for Antibiotics (OMA) model. *Globalization and Health*, *9*, 58. https://doi.org/10.1186/1744-8603-9-58

Cabral, C., Horwood, J., Hay, A. D., & Lucas, P. J. (2014). How communication affects prescription decisions in consultations for acute illness in children: A systematic review and meta-ethnography. *BMC Family Practice*, *15*, 63. https://doi.org/10.1186/1471-2296-15-63

Cabral, C., Horwood, J., Symonds, J., Ingram, J., Lucas, P. J., Redmond, N. M., Kai, J., Hay, A. D., & Barnes, R. K. (2019). Understanding the influence of parent-clinician communication on antibiotic prescribing for children with respiratory tract infections in primary care: A qualitative observational study using a conversation analysis approach. *BMC Family Practice*, *20*(1), 102. https://doi.org/10.1186/s12875-019-0993-9

CARSS. (2016). *C.A.R.S.S. China antimicrobial resistance surveillance system report 2015* (China Licensed Pharmacist 2016, Vol. 13, pp. 3–8). Committee of Experts on Rational Drug Use; National Health and Family Planning Commission of the P.R. China.

CDC. (2021, November 23). *The biggest antibiotic-resistant threats in the U.S.* Centers for Disease Control and Prevention. https://www.cdc.gov/drugresistance/biggest-threats.html

Chan, M. (2011, April 6). *WHO World Health Day 2011: Combat drug resistance: No action today means no cure tomorrow*. http://www.who.int/mediacentre/news/statements/2011/whd_20110407/en/

Currie, J., Lin, W., & Zhang, W. (2011). Patient knowledge and antibiotic abuse: Evidence from an audit study in China. *Journal of Health Economics*, *30*(5), 933–949. https://doi.org/10.1016/j.jhealeco.2011.05.009

Fleming-Dutra, K. E., Hersh, A. L., Shapiro, D. J., Bartoces, M., Enns, E. A., File, T. M., Finkelstein, J. A., Gerber, J. S., Hyun, D. Y., Linder, J. A., Lynfield, R., Margolis, D. J., May, L. S., Merenstein, D., Metlay, J. P., Newland, J. G., Piccirillo, J. F., Roberts, R. M., Sanchez, G. V., . . . Hicks, L. A. (2016). Prevalence of inappropriate antibiotic prescriptions among US ambulatory care visits, 2010–2011. *JAMA*, *315*(17), 1864–1873. https://doi.org/10.1001/jama.2016.4151

Fletcher-Lartey, S., Yee, M., Gaarslev, C., & Khan, R. (2016). Why do general practitioners prescribe antibiotics for upper respiratory tract infections to meet patient expectations: A mixed methods study. *BMJ Open*, *6*(10), e012244. https://doi.org/10.1136/bmjopen-2016-012244

He, A. J. (2014). The doctor–patient relationship, defensive medicine and overprescription in Chinese public hospitals: Evidence from a cross-sectional survey in Shenzhen city. *Social Science & Medicine*, *123*, 64–71. https://doi.org/10.1016/j.socscimed.2014.10.055

Heritage, J., Elliott, M. N., Stivers, T., Richardson, A., & Mangione-Smith, R. (2010). Reducing inappropriate antibiotics prescribing: The role of online commentary on physical examination findings. *Patient Education and Counseling*, *81*(1), 119–125. https://doi.org/10.1016/j.pec.2009.12.005

Heritage, J., & Stivers, T. (1999). Online commentary in acute medical visits: A method of shaping patient expectations. *Social Science & Medicine (1982)*, *49*(11), 1501–1517.

Hicks, L. A., Bartoces, M. G., Roberts, R. M., Suda, K. J., Hunkler, R. J., Taylor, T. H., & Schrag, S. J. (2015). US outpatient antibiotic prescribing variation according to geography, patient population, and provider specialty in 2011. *Clinical Infectious Diseases: An Official Publication of the Infectious Diseases Society of America*, *60*(9), 1308–1316. https://doi.org/10.1093/cid/civ076

Horton, R. (2019). Offline: AMR – The end of modern medicine? *The Lancet*, *393*(10172), 624. https://doi.org/10.1016/S0140-6736(19)30367-8

Kronman, M. P., Gerber, J. S., Grundmeier, R. W., Zhou, C., Robinson, J. D., Heritage, J., Stout, J., Burges, D., Hedrick, B., Warren, L., Shalowitz, M., Shone, L. P., Steffes, J., Wright, M., Fiks, A. G., & Mangione-Smith, R. (2020). Reducing antibiotic prescribing in primary care for respiratory illness. *Pediatrics, 146*(3). https://doi.org/10.1542/peds.2020-0038

Kumar, S., Little, P., & Britten, N. (2003). Why do general practitioners prescribe antibiotics for sore throat? Grounded theory interview study. *BMJ: British Medical Journal, 326*(7381), 138.

Laxminarayan, R., Duse, A., Wattal, C., Zaidi, A. K. M., Wertheim, H. F. L., Sumpradit, N., Vlieghe, E., Hara, G. L., Gould, I. M., Goossens, H., Greko, C., So, A. D., Bigdeli, M., Tomson, G., Woodhouse, W., Ombaka, E., Peralta, A. Q., Qamar, F. N., Mir, F., . . . Cars, O. (2013a). Antibiotic resistance-the need for global solutions. *The Lancet. Infectious Diseases, 13*(12), 1057–1098. https://doi.org/10.1016/S1473-3099(13)70318-9

Laxminarayan, R., Duse, A., Wattal, C., Zaidi, A. K. M., Wertheim, H. F. L., Sumpradit, N., Vlieghe, E., Hara, G. L., Gould, I. M., Goossens, H., Greko, C., So, A. D., Bigdeli, M., Tomson, G., Woodhouse, W., Ombaka, E., Peralta, A. Q., Qamar, F. N., Mir, F., . . . Cars, O. (2013b). Antibiotic resistance-the need for global solutions. *The Lancet. Infectious Diseases, 13*(12), 1057–1098. https://doi.org/10.1016/S1473-3099(13)70318-9

Laxminarayan, R., Matsoso, P., Pant, S., Brower, C., Røttingen, J.-A., Klugman, K., & Davies, S. (2016). Access to effective antimicrobials: A worldwide challenge. *Lancet (London, England), 387*(10014), 168–175. https://doi.org/10.1016/S0140-6736(15)00474-2

Li, Y., Xu, J., Wang, F., Wang, B., Liu, L., Hou, W., Fan, H., Tong, Y., Zhang, J., & Lu, Z. (2012). Overprescribing in China, driven by financial incentives, results in very high use of antibiotics, injections, and corticosteroids. *Health Affairs, 31*(5), 1075–1082. https://doi.org/10.1377/hlthaff.2010.0965

Linder, J. A., & Singer, D. E. (2003). Desire for antibiotics and antibiotic prescribing for adults with upper respiratory tract infections. *Journal of General Internal Medicine, 18*(10), 795–801. https://doi.org/10.1046/j.1525-1497.2003.21101.x

Mangione-Smith, R., Elliott, M. N., Stivers, T., McDonald, L. L., & Heritage, J. (2006). Ruling out the need for antibiotics: Are we sending the right message? *Archives of Pediatrics & Adolescent Medicine, 160*(9), 945–952. https://doi.org/10.1001/archpedi.160.9.945

Mangione-Smith, R., McGlynn, E., Elliott, M. N., Krogstad, P., & Brook, R. H. (1999). The relationship between perceived parental expectations and pediatrician antimicrobial prescribing behavior. *Pediatrics, 103*(4), 711–718.

Mangione-Smith, R., McGlynn, E., Elliott, N., McDonald, L., Franz, L., & Kravitz, L. (2001). Parent expectations for antibiotics, physician-parent communication, and satisfaction. *Archives of Pediatrics and Adolescent Medicine, 155*(7), 800–806.

Mei, Y., & Tong, M. (2012). Mohnarin annual report 2010: Surveillance of antibiotic resistance in bacteria isolated from young adults. *Chinese Journal of Nosocomiology*. https://www.semanticscholar.org/paper/Mohnarin-annual-report-2010%3Asurveillance-of-in-from-Ming-qing/710c55cf0ac7b6d58ff004cfffe2d46fe31c396f

Mölstad, S., Erntell, M., Hanberger, H., Melander, E., Norman, C., Skoog, G., Lundborg, C., Söderström, A., Torell, E., & Cars, O. (2008). Sustained reduction of antibiotic use and low bacterial resistance: 10-year follow-up of the Swedish Strama programme – The lancet infectious diseases. *The Lancet Infectious Diseases, 8*(2), 125–132. https://doi.org10.1016/S1473-3099(08)70017-3

Murray, C. J., Ikuta, K. S., Sharara, F., Swetschinski, L., Aguilar, G. R., Gray, A., Han, C., Bisignano, C., Rao, P., Wool, E., Johnson, S. C., Browne, A. J., Chipeta, M. G., Fell, F.,

Hackett, S., Haines-Woodhouse, G., Hamadani, B. H. K., Kumaran, E. A. P., McManigal, B., . . . Naghavi, M. (2022). Global burden of bacterial antimicrobial resistance in 2019: A systematic analysis. *The Lancet*, *399*(10325), 629–655. https://doi.org/10.1016/S0140-6736(21)02724-0

Nowakowska, M., van Staa, T., Mölter, A., Ashcroft, D. M., Tsang, J. Y., White, A., Welfare, W., & Palin, V. (2019). Antibiotic choice in UK general practice: Rates and drivers of potentially inappropriate antibiotic prescribing. *The Journal of Antimicrobial Chemotherapy*, *74*(11), 3371–3378. https://doi.org/10.1093/jac/dkz345

O'Connor, R., O'Doherty, J., O'Regan, A., & Dunne, C. (2018). Antibiotic use for acute respiratory tract infections (ARTI) in primary care; what factors affect prescribing and why is it important? A narrative review. *Irish Journal of Medical Science (1971-)*, *187*(4), 969–986. https://doi.org/10.1007/s11845-018-1774-5

O'Neil, J. (2015). *Antimicrobial resistance: Tackling a crisis for the health and wealth of nations/the review on antimicrobial resistance chaired by Jim O'Neill. (review on antimicrobial resistance, 2015.)*. https://wellcomecollection.org/works/rdpck35v

Ong, S., Nakase, J., Moran, G. J., Karras, D. J., Kuehnert, M. J., Talan, D. A., & EMERGEncy ID NET Study Group. (2007). Antibiotic use for emergency department patients with upper respiratory infections: Prescribing practices, patient expectations, and patient satisfaction. *Annals of Emergency Medicine*, *50*(3), 213–220. https://doi.org/10.1016/j.annemergmed.2007.03.026

Reynolds, L., & Mckee, M. (2009). Factors influencing antibiotic prescribing in China: An exploratory analysis. *Health Policy*, *90*(1), 32–36.

Sabuncu, E., David, J., Bernède-Bauduin, C., Pépin, S., Leroy, M., Boëlle, P.-Y., Watier, L., & Guillemot, D. (2009). Significant reduction of antibiotic use in the community after a nationwide campaign in France, 2002–2007. *PLoS Medicine*, *6*(6), e1000084. https://doi.org/10.1371/journal.pmed.1000084

Scott, J. G., Cohen, D., DiCicco-Bloom, B., Orzano, A. J., Jaen, C. R., & Crabtree, B. F. (2001). Antibiotic use in acute respiratory infections and the ways patients pressure physicians for a prescription. *The Journal of Family Practice*, *50*(10), 853–858.

Shlaes, D. M., Sahm, D., Opiela, C., & Spellberg, B. (2013). The FDA reboot of antibiotic development. *Antimicrobial Agents and Chemotherapy*, *57*(10), 4605–4607. https://doi.org/10.1128/AAC.01277-13

Stivers, T. (2002a). Participating in decisions about treatment: Overt parent pressure for antibiotic medication in pediatric encounters. *Social Science & Medicine*, *54*(7), 1111–1130.

Stivers, T. (2002b). "Symptoms only" and "Candidate diagnoses": Presenting the problem in pediatric encounters. *Health Communication*, *3*(14), 299–338.

Stivers, T. (2005). Parent resistance to physicians' treatment recommendations: One resource for initiating a negotiation of the treatment decision. *Health Communication*, *181*(1), 41–74.

Stivers, T. (2007). *Prescribing under pressure: Physician-parent conversations and antibiotics*. Oxford University Press.

Stivers, T., & Timmermans, S. (2020). Medical authority under siege: How clinicians transform patient resistance into acceptance. *Journal of Health and Social Behavior*, *61*(1), 60–78. https://doi.org/10.1177/0022146520902740

Stivers, T., & Timmermans, S. (2021). Arriving at no: Patient pressure to prescribe antibiotics and physicians' responses. *Social Science & Medicine*, *290*, 114007. https://doi.org/10.1016/j.socscimed.2021.114007

Wang, J., Wang, P., Wang, X., Zheng, Y., & Xiao, Y. (2014). Use and prescription of antibiotics in primary health care settings in China. *JAMA Internal Medicine*, *174*(12), 1914–1920. https://doi.org/10.1001/jamainternmed.2014.5214

Wang, N. C. (2020). Understanding antibiotic overprescribing in China: A conversation analysis approach. *Social Science & Medicine*, *262*, 113251. https://doi.org/10.1016/j.socscimed.2020.113251

Wang, N. C., & Liu, Y. (2021). Going shopping or consulting in medical visits: Caregivers' roles in pediatric antibiotic prescribing in China. *Social Science & Medicine*, 114075. https://doi.org/10.1016/j.socscimed.2021.114075

Wang, S. Y., Cantarelli, P., Groene, O., Stargardt, T., & Belle, N. (2023). Patient expectations do matter – Experimental evidence on antibiotic prescribing decisions among hospital-based physicians. *Health Policy*, *128*, 11–17. https://doi.org/10.1016/j.healthpol.2022.11.009

WHO. (2014). *Antimicrobial resistance: Global report on surveillance 2014 (194; antimicrobial resistance)*. http://www.who.int/mediacentre/factsheets/fs194/en/

WHO. (2020a). *Antimicrobial resistance (antimicrobial resistance) [World Health Organization Fact Sheets]*. World Health Organization. https://www.who.int/news-room/fact-sheets/detail/antimicrobial-resistance

WHO. (2020b, July 31). *Antibiotic resistance* [Fact Sheet]. https://www.who.int/news-room/fact-sheets/detail/antibiotic-resistance

Xiao, Y., Wang, J., Li, Y., & MOH National Antimicrobial Resistance Investigation Net. (2008). Bacterial resistance surveillance in China: A report from Mohnarin 2004–2005. *European Journal of Clinical Microbiology & Infectious Diseases*, *27*(8), 697–708.

Yip, W., Powell-Jackson, T., Chen, W., Hu, M., Fe, E., Hu, M., Jian, W., Lu, M., Han, W., & Hsiao, W. C. (2014). Capitation combined with pay-for-performance improves antibiotic prescribing practices in rural China. *Health Affairs*. https://doi.org/10.1377/hlthaff.2013.0702

Zhang, Q.-Q., Ying, G.-G., Pan, C.-G., Liu, Y.-S., & Zhao, J.-L. (2015). Comprehensive evaluation of antibiotics emission and fate in the river basins of China: Source analysis, multimedia modeling, and linkage to bacterial resistance. *Environmental Science & Technology*, *49*(11), 6772–6782. https://doi.org/10.1021/acs.est.5b00729

Zhao, H., Bian, J., Han, X., Zhang, M., & Zhan, S. (2020). Outpatient antibiotic use associated with acute upper respiratory infections in China: A nationwide cross-sectional study. *International Journal of Antimicrobial Agents*, *56*(6), 106193. https://doi.org/10.1016/j.ijantimicag.2020.106193

Zhao, H., Wei, L., Li, H., Zhang, M., Cao, B., Bian, J., & Zhan, S. (2021). Appropriateness of antibiotic prescriptions in ambulatory care in China: A nationwide descriptive database study. *Lancet Infect Dis*. 2021 Jun; *21*(6):847–857. doi: 10.1016/S1473-3099(20)30596-X. Epub 2021 Jan 27. PMID: 33515511.

2 Historical and institutional factors of antibiotic overprescription in China

Introduction

Institutional factors related to the historical transformations of Chinese society and its healthcare system have been identified as the most significant contributors to the problem of antibiotic overprescription. For a relatively extended period (from the late 1980s to the early 2010s), doctors were blamed for prescribing more antibiotics than necessary, driven by financial incentives tied to their prescriptions. These perverse incentives were created at both individual and organizational levels and reinforced by a complex matrix of stakeholders, making doctors the primary target for addressing the antibiotic overprescription problem.

Despite the general acceptance of supply-side related theories, the complexity of the problem of antibiotic overprescription in China has been largely overlooked. If the problem were solely driven by financial incentives tied to doctors' prescriptions, one would expect it to be easily solved by removing the perverse incentives. However, the problem persists despite substantial efforts and resources directed toward addressing it from the supply side. These efforts include policy changes that remove perverse incentives, reforms to providers' payment schemes, and sanction measures under a strict antibiotic stewardship program. Yet, antibiotic prescription rates remain high.

What complexity might be involved in the problem? What factors might have been overlooked in understanding the problem? How are the historical and institutional factors related to these missing variables? In this chapter, I aim to provide a synthesized overview of the historical and institutional factors that existing research has identified as contributing to the problem. Apart from contextualizing the main findings of the book, it is also my goal to argue that these historical and institutional factors no longer directly drive the problem by creating perverse incentives for doctors. Rather, they exert a more subtle influence by shaping a medical culture that relies heavily on antibiotics and indirectly affecting patients' health-seeking behavior and attitudes toward antibiotics in their everyday lives.

A typical medical encounter

On an ordinary autumn day, Tian's mother notices that he has a slight cough. Although the cough is mild, its presence causes her to worry. Last autumn, Tian had a similar condition that later turned into pneumonia and kept Tian and his

DOI: 10.4324/9781003243625-2

mother hospitalized for 15 days. To prevent this from happening again, she buys a pack of oral antibiotics at a nearby pharmacy. After using it for two days, the cough persists. The next day, she brings Tian to visit a doctor at the local hospital:

> *Upon entering the consultation room, Tian and his mother found that the doctor was still with the previous patient. When that patient left, they quickly presented Tian's problem to the doctor. The consultation did not last long, and the doctor recommended a non-antibiotic oral treatment. However, this non-antibiotic recommendation is resisted by Tian's mother. Instead, she requested an antibiotic IV infusion. Having already tried the most expensive oral antibiotic before they came in, she did not believe that any oral medication would work. Despite the doctor's efforts to persuade her, she insisted on receiving an antibiotic IV infusion, and the doctor ultimately agreed.*

This is a typical scenario in the pediatric outpatient care setting where the book's study is situated. On average, these medical encounters last around five minutes. Some are even shorter, with caregivers coming in only for specific prescriptions. Others are longer, with doctors and caregivers engaging in extended discussions about treatment decisions. Regardless of their length, these consultations share some common contextual features: a fast-paced environment, overloaded hospitals, overworked doctors, long waits, and a tension-filled doctor–patient relationship.

These contextual features not only set the scene for the book's findings but are also related to the historical and institutional factors that the existing literature has identified as contributing to the problem of antibiotic overprescription in China. Next, I will provide a concise introduction to the organization of the healthcare system, aiming to give readers a general sense of what it is like to seek care in China. I will then discuss briefly how these historical and institutional factors contribute to the rampant antibiotic overprescription problem by creating a complex matrix of perverse incentives and shaping an antibiotic-saturated medical culture.

The healthcare system

History: healthcare system in the Mao era (1949–1978)

China's healthcare system made significant achievements during the Mao era. Prior to 1949, the health status of the Chinese population was among the worst in the world. However, during the Mao era, the average life expectancy rose from 35 to 68, and infant mortality fell from 250 to 40 deaths per 1,000 births (Hsiao, 1995). Despite low standards of care – 'barefoot doctors' who provided basic health services in rural areas had only a few months of training after secondary school – widespread availability and use of basic medicines and an emphasis on controlling infectious diseases helped improve the country's health status, achieving "the most rapid sustained increase in documented global history" (Eggleston, 2012).

The healthcare system during this era was characterized by central planning, with an emphasis on 'prevention first,' community organization, and cooperative financing (Hsiao, 1995). Under this system, the rural population was covered by the Cooperative Medical Scheme (CMS), with village doctors providing primary care and being employed and paid by commune health stations. In urban areas, the growing urban population was largely covered by two types of insurance programs – the Government Insurance Scheme (GIS) and the Labor Insurance Scheme (LIS). The GIS, financed by government budgets, provided healthcare service to government employees, retirees, disabled veterans, and university students, while the LIS, financed by each enterprise's welfare fund, provided healthcare services to state enterprise employees, their dependents, and retirees (Yip & Hsiao, 2008).

Overall, during this era, almost the entire Chinese population had insurance coverage, healthcare services were paid for through social insurance programs, and patients' out-of-pocket payments were minimal. It is widely recognized that the healthcare system achieved enviable success in improving the Chinese population's health status during the Mao era (Eggleston, 2012).

Present: healthcare system in post-Mao era (1979 to now)

With the social and economic reforms that began in 1979, the healthcare system underwent significant transformation. Over the three decades since, the majority of the population lost insurance, medical services became less affordable, and the public became vulnerable to adverse medical consequences (Eggleston, 2012). These transformations had significant consequences on the problem of antibiotic overprescription in China. In the following, I briefly explain the organization of the healthcare system, aiming to show: Where do patients go when they are ill? What kind of healthcare service do they receive? What kind of doctor–patient relationship do they have?

Leadership and financing – the public hospital system

Healthcare institutions are mostly public, either directly or indirectly owned by the state. Statistics in 2011 showed that 62% of hospitals are public and 38% are private (Wu et al., 2013). In terms of market share, public hospitals provided 91% of the total service provision volume, while private hospitals (including private clinics) only accounted for 9% of all services provided. In terms of function, most public hospitals are general-acute hospitals; private hospitals are usually smaller, specialized, and less likely to be included in the social insurance system, such as orthopedic hospitals, eye hospitals, or dental hospitals.

Private hospitals have to compete with public hospitals for location, services offered, and prices charged. Despite their relatively low status, the number of private hospitals has been increasing as the central government opened up the healthcare services market to private investment more recently. According to a market report, there were 15,798 private hospitals in 2016, accounting for 55.3% of the total hospitals. However, the revenue of private hospitals was less than 10% of the total hospital revenue (Wu et al., 2013). That is to say, hospitals or institutions in China are mostly public and provide the majority of the healthcare services.

Service delivery and hospital – the three-tier system

Generally, rural residents rely on a three-tier clinic-based service delivery network for their healthcare needs, while urban residents mostly rely on a three-tier hospital-based service delivery system (Yip et al., 2010). Village health clinics and community health centers provide basic primary care to rural and urban residents, respectively; township health centers and county hospitals provide rural patients with referral services and receive patients with greater medical needs. In urban areas, secondary hospitals and tertiary hospitals provide patients with more comprehensive medical services. Public health organizations are supplemental to the three-tier service network in both rural and urban areas.

HEALTHCARE SERVICES IN RURAL AREAS

In rural areas, a three-tier health service delivery network was established, with each tier operating at a different administrative level. On top are the county hospitals (including traditional Chinese medicine hospitals), followed by township health centers and then village clinics. The three-tier network provides rural residents with basic health services such as primary care, prevention, health inspection, and health education (The State Council Information Office, China, 2012).

The three-tier health service delivery network is also designed with a referral system. Rural residents are supposed to go to village clinics, the first tier, for primary care and basic health services. If the problems need a higher level of care, patients are referred to a nearby township health center – the second tier. Services provided in township health centers include delivering babies, treating infections and wounds, and minor surgeries such as appendectomies. County hospitals – the third tier – are the last point of referral for inpatient treatment as well as a wide range of services (Eggleston, 2012; Hsiao, 1997).

Despite the fact that the three-tier network and the referral system were established to solve patients' health problems, mostly in township health centers and village clinics, it has been found that township health centers do not receive many patients. Studies show that rural residents (1) tend to leave their health problems unattended, (2) tend to visit village clinics more frequently than township health centers, and (3) tend to bypass township health centers and go directly to county hospitals when having major health problems despite long travel times and high transportation costs (Liu et al., 2007).

HEALTHCARE SERVICES IN URBAN AREAS

In urban areas, hospitals are organized in a three-tier scheme, providing primary and a wide range of specialized healthcare services. The classification is mainly based on scale (bed and staff number), coverage region, and service provision. The tertiary hospitals, on the top of the tier system, are the fewest in number but have the most resources. Tertiary hospitals are equipped with over 500 beds and are responsible for providing high-standard and specialized medical services across regions, provinces, and nationwide. They are also responsible for providing technical guidance to lower-level hospitals. Secondary hospitals are regional hospitals. They are equipped with 100–500 beds and provide general medical services to multiple communities in one region. Primary hospitals – at the bottom of the tier system – are the greatest in number, cover a single community, and have the fewest resources. They are equipped with 20–100 beds and are responsible for primary care as well as preventative and rehabilitation services in a single community.

With the three-tier hospital-based system, urban residents are supposed to follow a referral system for their medical visits. They visit primary hospitals in their community for prevention, rehabilitation services, and primary care for common and minor health conditions. Patients with major health conditions should be referred to regional secondary hospitals. Patients with unresolved and severe conditions should then be referred to tertiary hospitals for higher-standard care and specialized care. Yet, this is not the case in reality.

Although the abovementioned referral system exists and the social health insurance programs limit coverage for healthcare services outside patients' given locality (county and municipality), patients are free to choose whichever level of hospital they wish and can pay for. The hospital referral system is considered to exist in name only. This results in the overloading of outpatient service departments in tertiary and secondary hospitals (Li & Xie, 2013), a major problem in the current urban healthcare service delivery system. A small number of hospitals, especially the tertiary hospitals in metro cities, serve a disproportionate volume of patients, including for minor conditions. The resultant high-level occupational stress among doctors is significantly associated with doctors' low perceived professional efficacy, dissatisfaction with the doctor–patient relationship, high over-commitment, low decision authority, and low skill discretion (Wu et al., 2013).

Services are disproportionately provided across different tiers of hospitals. Tertiary hospitals constitute 10% of all hospitals but provide 38% of all outpatient services and 36% of all inpatient services. In comparison, primary hospitals comprise 42% of hospitals, but their service provision is much less than that of tertiary hospitals – 10% of outpatient services and 5% of inpatient services.

A ubiquitous slogan that captures the average urban Chinese patient's concern about access to appropriate and high-quality care is *kan bing nan, kan bing gui* (getting health care is difficult, and getting health care is expensive), as they have to wait longer, communicate less, and pay more, especially when seeking care in the overwhelmingly overloaded hospital environment.

These structural issues relating to the organization of the healthcare system are argued as primarily attributable to the antibiotic overprescription problem. In the following, I show a matrix of perverse incentives created at different levels, collectively contributing to the antibiotic overprescription problem in Chinese clinical settings.

Perverse incentives at the hospital level

Public hospitals dominate China's healthcare system, yet they only receive minimal funding support from the government. Thus, they have to rely on drug sales for survival. As mentioned earlier, public hospitals account for 62% of health institutions in China, and they provide 91% of the healthcare services (Wu et al., 2013); however, after the country embarked on market reforms in 1979, the central government reduced subsidies to public hospitals from more than 50% to about 10% (Eggleston, 2012). As a result, user fees and drug sales have become a major source of revenue for public hospitals to survive financially. It was estimated that drug sales accounted for over half of hospital revenues, with antibiotics accounting for 47% of all drug sales (Yip et al., 2010).

Moreover, a 15% markup policy for hospital drug sales has been in place for at least two decades since the market reforms in 1979, which has further influenced providers' prescribing behaviors over the past three decades. To ensure that basic health services remain affordable even for the poor, the government set prices for these services below cost; however, it allowed a 15% profit margin for drugs prescribed and set the prices for new and high-technology diagnostic services above cost (Yip et al., 2010). These pricing policies, thus, caused an erosion of professional medical ethics, and overprescription driven by financial profit has become widespread in China (Li et al., 2012; Yip et al., 2010).

A famous slogan, *yi yao yang yi* (hospitals and doctors rely on drug sales for survival), characterizes this problem. Prescribing for profit has been recognized as a remarkable problem in the healthcare system, contributing to rising medical expenses, patient distrust, and overprescription of drugs in China (Zhu, 2012). It is found that drug expenditures account for 45% of health expenditures on average – the highest in the world; also, the sales volume of drugs is positively associated with drug price – the higher a drug's price, the more it is sold.

Perverse incentives at the doctor level

Similar to the situation in hospitals, doctors, as employees of public hospitals, also rely on drug sales for survival (Zhu, 2012). The basic salaries of health providers in public hospitals have remained low, similar to those of government staff according to their professional rank and length of service. A survey conducted by a renowned online forum for health providers reported that 75% of respondents had an annual income of less than RMB 40,000 (around USD $6,452) – less than RMB 3,300 (USD $524) monthly (Global Times, 2009). Despite the increase in average individual income across economic sectors, as well as the fast increase in the per capita GDP over the past three decades, the income of doctors has not changed much over the years, and it ranks behind the income levels of many other sectors such as IT, finance, scientific research, entertainment, and logistics (Global Times, 2009).

Furthermore, to ensure that healthcare services are accessible to everyone, particularly those with low incomes, the government has set the price of doctor consultations extremely low, at around RMB 2 (USD 30 cents) per visit. Consequently, hospitals and doctors struggle to sustain themselves on this income alone. In order to generate profits to fund expansions in bed capacity and technology, doctors are encouraged to prescribe more medication (Yip et al., 2010). Consequently, a greater proportion of their income comes from sources other than their basic salary.

A major source of income for doctors is performance pay, which is determined by the amount of profits generated by the doctors, primarily through drug sales. Performance pay accounts for a large proportion of the providers' income, sometimes 3–8 times their basic salary, though this varies by doctors' rank, type of clinic, and geographic location. Although there is no data on how much doctors can earn through performance pay, a regulation put forward by the Shenzhen municipal government on hospital performance pay in 2012 can provide us with some insight. This policy stipulates that the performance pay of hospital leaders cannot exceed 300% of the average income of all hospital employees, the performance pay of hospital deputy leaders cannot exceed 200% of the average income of all hospital employees, and the performance pay of a clinic department director cannot exceed 150% of the average income of all hospital employees (Zhu, 2012).

Perverse incentives from the pharmaceutical industry

Commissions or bonuses provided by pharmaceutical companies are also a regular source of income for doctors. This part of income can be 2–3 times a doctor's basic salary and can vary by the type of doctor and drug (Zhu, 2012). As mentioned previously, both hospitals and doctors rely on drug prescriptions as a major source of income that is important for their own survival. It is widely acknowledged that hospitals regularly receive 'kickbacks,' and doctors receive 'bonuses' from pharmaceutical businesses for prescribing their products (W. Yip & Hsiao, 2008). Together, such practices by pharmaceutical companies create further financial incentives for overprescription.

Kickbacks paid to hospitals take various forms. On the first level, public hospitals, given their monopoly position in the healthcare service provision market, are able to collaborate with pharmaceutical businesses to set a nominal purchase price that is several times higher than its factory price for certain drugs (Zhu, 2012). The following example illustrates how such kickbacks work:

> *If the actual factory price of a medicine is $2, with the 15% markup, $0.30 cents can be added to the retail price of the medicine sold at the hospital, and it can be kept by the hospital as profit. However, if the hospital and the pharmaceutical business agree to set the purchasing price at $20 instead of $2, $3 can be added to the retail price legally as profit. Furthermore, pharmaceutical businesses will give the $18 margin to the hospital as a kickback. In this case, the hospital gains $21 in total as profit (this amount partially goes to hospital administrators and partially to individual doctors). The pharmaceutical kickbacks to hospitals can take an even more subtle form. For example, some pharmaceutical businesses allow hospitals to pay what they owe 6–12 months later. This becomes an invisible loan to hospitals at zero interest.*
>
> (Zhu, 2012)

On the individual doctor level, besides providing monetary kickbacks as mentioned, pharmaceutical businesses also conduct "rebating" practices, including organizing conference tours, buying lunches and beverages for doctors during their busy schedule, and offering gifts, practices similar to those described in *Medicine, Money, and Morals* regarding doctors' conflicts of interest in the United States (Rodwin, 1993).

In sum, the business practices of pharmaceutical companies strengthen the financial incentives for the overprescription of drugs both at the institutional level and the individual level. With little monitoring or regulation at the organizational level to oversee hospitals' or doctors' practices and conflicts of interest, overprescription driven by financial incentives is widespread.

Other structural factors: lower qualifications of health providers in rural areas

The simple fact that health professionals are insufficiently trained also contributes to the overprescription problem. Studies show that the overprovision of drugs is rampant in rural China, alongside the provision of expired and counterfeit drugs. The problem of low-skilled and low-quality health professionals is particularly severe in rural areas (Yip et al., 2010). In rural areas, residents receive far lower quality healthcare services compared to urban residents. Studies show that 70% of providers have achieved less than a high school degree and have received only 20 months of medical training on average (Eggleston et al., 2008; Wang & He, 2003). Some providers rely half on their medical practice and half on farming to make their living (Hsiao, 1997).

In addition, the service quality of county hospitals, which are considered the highest level for rural residents, is not as good as that of average hospitals in urban areas. Researchers conducted a study in four township health centers and eight village health clinics in Chongqing and Gansu and found that less than 2% of drug prescriptions were 'rational' in township health centers and village clinics, and only 0.06% of drug prescriptions in village clinics were reasonable (Wang & He, 2003).

The matrix of institutional factors, including insufficient funding support from the government, low compensation for healthcare providers, unregulated business practices of pharmaceutical companies, and low qualifications of rural healthcare providers, have all been shown to contribute to antibiotic overprescribing in China. These historical and institutional factors have directly influenced doctors' prescribing behaviors for an extended period. Even after the perverse incentives are removed, they continue to exert their influence in a more subtle and indirect manner.

A spillover effect: An antibiotic-saturated medical culture

Following the supply-side theory, major policy changes have been initiated to address the issue. For example, a 'zero markup' policy has replaced the old '15% markup' drug policy since 2009, removing the perverse incentive tied to doctors' prescribing. Serious antibiotic stewardship programs were launched in selected hospitals in 2012, monitoring and regulating doctors' antibiotic prescriptions by sanctioning overprescription (e.g., suspension of professional licenses, removal from post (Wang et al., 2016; Xiao et al., 2013)). However, the effects of these measures have been less than satisfactory (Wang et al., 2020; Wang et al., 2014; Xiao, 2018).

Then, what is missing from our understanding of the antibiotic overprescription problem? Apart from the direct effects of these historical and institutional factors on the problem, this book argues that they also indirectly influence by creating an antibiotic-saturated medical culture. This medical culture subtly shapes patients' and caregivers' health-seeking behaviors and attitudes toward antibiotics. Antibiotics are taken for granted for even self-limiting and inappropriate conditions. With easy access in the retail market, they are treated like Mentos candy that can be easily purchased without a doctor's prescription. In medical encounters, patients orient themselves as entitled to negotiate for antibiotic prescriptions, including those for restricted use and in more invasive forms of administration (e.g., intravenous or intramuscular injections).

Conclusion

Perhaps the most discussed contributing factors to China's antibiotic overprescription problem are the institutional or structural factors relating to the transformation of the healthcare system. The institutional factors, specifically how the healthcare system is organized – its governance, financing structure, service delivery system, and its relation to doctors' prescriptions, indeed, have an effect that is nonnegligible and far-reaching.

However, the institutional factors at the macro-level alone do not explain the continuation and even exacerbation of the antibiotic overprescription problem in China. In the following chapters, I will first present findings from a national survey, showing the pre-visit self-medication behavior and expectations for antibiotics as well as their relationship with the prescriptions they receive during the medical visits. I will then move our attention to the interaction process within the clinical encounters, where antibiotic prescribing decisions are made interactionally and collaboratively between doctors and patient caregivers.

References

Eggleston, K. (2012). *Health care for 1.3 billion: An overview of China's health system (SSRN scholarly paper ID 2029952)*. Social Science Research Network. http://papers. ssrn.com/abstract=2029952

Eggleston, K., Ling, L., Qingyue, M., Lindelow, M., & Wagstaff, A. (2008). Health service delivery in China: A literature review. *Health Economics*, *17*(2), 149–165. https://doi. org/10.1002/hec.1306

Global Times. (2009). Is providers' income low: How much do providers earn? *Global Times*. http://www.med126.com/news/2009/20090402221858_108589.shtml

Hsiao, W.C. (1997). *Financing health care: Issues and options for China* (Vol. 17091, pp. 1–84). The World Bank. http://documents.worldbank.org/curated/en/1997/09/12638366/ financing-health-care-issues-options-china

Hsiao, W. C. (1995). The Chinese health care system: Lessons for other nations. *Social Science & Medicine (1982), 41*(8), 1047–1055.

Li, Q., & Xie, P. (2013). Outpatient workload in China. *Lancet, 381*(9882), 1983–1984. https://doi.org/10.1016/S0140-6736(13)61198-8

Li, Y., Xu, J., Wang, F., Wang, B., Liu, L., Hou, W., Fan, H., Tong, Y., Zhang, J., & Lu, Z. (2012). Overprescribing in China, driven by financial incentives, results in very high use of antibiotics, injections, and corticosteroids. *Health Affairs, 31*(5), 1075–1082. https://doi.org/10.1377/hlthaff.2010.0965

Liu, M., Zhang, Q., Lu, M., Kwon, C.-S., & Quan, H. (2007). Rural and urban disparity in health services utilization in China. *Medical Care, 45*(8), 767–774. https://doi.org/10.1097/MLR.0b013e3180618b9a

Rodwin, M. (1993). *Medicine, money, and morals: Physicians' conflicts of interests.* Oxford University Press.

The State Council Information Office, China. (2012). *White paper: Medical and health services in China.* http://www.scio.gov.cn/ztk/dtzt/91/12/Document/1262955/1262955.htm

Wang, C., Huttner, B. D., Magrini, N., Cheng, Y., Tong, J., Li, S., Wan, C., Zhu, Q., Zhao, S., Zhuo, Z., Lin, D., Yi, B., Shan, Q., Long, M., Jia, C., Zhao, D., Sun, X., Liu, J., Zhou, Y., . . . Hu, H. (2020). Pediatric antibiotic prescribing in China according to the 2019 World Health Organization Access, Watch, and Reserve (AWaRe) antibiotic categories. *The Journal of Pediatrics, 220*, 125–131.e5. https://doi.org/10.1016/j.jpeds.2020.01.044

Wang, J., Wang, P., Wang, X., Zheng, Y., & Xiao, Y. (2014). Use and prescription of antibiotics in primary health care settings in China. *JAMA Internal Medicine, 174*(12), 1914–1920. https://doi.org/10.1001/jamainternmed.2014.5214

Wang, L., Zhang, X., Liang, X., & Bloom, G. (2016). Addressing antimicrobial resistance in China: Policy implementation in a complex context. *Globalization and Health, 12*, 30. https://doi.org/10.1186/s12992-016-0167-7

Wang, Z., & He, S. (2003). Why NCMS in Wuxue can be sustained and developed. *Chinese Rural Health Care Management, 2*, 25–26.

Wu, C., Tian, Y., & Wong, J. (2013). *Investing in China hospital market.* Boston Consulting Group Publication.

Xiao, Y. (2018). Antimicrobial stewardship in China: Systems, actions and future strategies. *Clinical Infectious Diseases, 67*(suppl_2), S135–S141. https://doi.org/10.1093/cid/ciy641

Xiao, Y., Zhang, J., Zheng, B., Zhao, L., Li, S., & Li, L. (2013). Changes in Chinese policies to promote the rational use of antibiotics. *PLoS Medicine, 10*(11), e1001556. https://doi.org/10.1371/journal.pmed.1001556

Yip, W. C.-M., & Hsiao, W. C. (2008). The Chinese health system at a crossroads. *Health Affairs (Project Hope), 27*(2), 460–468. https://doi.org/10.1377/hlthaff.27.2.460

Yip, W. C.-M., Hsiao, W. C., Meng, Q., Chen, W., & Sun, X. (2010). Realignment of incentives for health-care providers in China. *The Lancet, 375*(9720), 1120–1130. https://doi.org/10.1016/S0140-6736(10)60063-3

Zhu, H. (2012). *Po Chu "Yi Yao Yang Yi" Ru He Ke Neng?* [Research paper]. http://ie.cass.cn/yjlw/01.asp?id=857

3 Outside the medical visit

Pre-visit use of non-prescribed
antibiotics, desires for antibiotic
prescriptions, and association with
antibiotic prescriptions in medical visits

Introduction

In Chapter 2, I discussed the historical and institutional factors that the existing literature identified as attributable to the antibiotic overprescription problem in China. I argued that these historical and institutional factors no longer contribute to the problem by directly driving doctors' prescriptions with perverse incentives; instead, they influence the problem subtly by creating a medical culture and shaping patients' and caregivers' behaviors and attitudes related to antibiotics when they manage common health conditions.

Considering the patients' or caregivers' expectations are cited by doctors as the most common reason for inappropriate prescription, it is thus relevant to ask: Is the antibiotic overprescription problem also influenced by patient caregivers' expectations? Moreover, self-medication, particularly the use of non-prescribed antibiotics, has been found to be a significant patient-related factor to the AMR pervasively observed in Asian countries. When patient caregivers' use of non-prescribed antibiotics fails, it is plausible that they would expect stronger or more advanced forms of treatment when they visit doctors.

In this chapter, I will present findings from a national survey examining the prevalence of patient caregivers' pre-visit use of non-prescribed antibiotics, their desires for antibiotics, the prescriptions they receive in the medical visit, and the relationships between them. In other words, I aim to answer the following questions: Do patient caregivers commonly use non-prescribed antibiotics when they manage their children's common cold symptoms? Do they frequently expect antibiotic prescriptions when they bring their children to visit doctors? Is there any association between caregivers' pre-visit use of non-prescribed antibiotics and the prescriptions that they receive during the medical visit? Relatedly, is there any association between caregivers' pre-visit expectations for antibiotics and the prescriptions that they receive in the medical visit? Lastly, I will discuss the predictors of caregivers' use of non-prescribed antibiotics and expectations for antibiotic prescriptions before medical visits.

Background

Patient-related factors such as self-medication have been identified by the WHO as one of the important contributors to inappropriate use of antibiotics (*WHO*

DOI: 10.4324/9781003243625-3

Global Strategy for Containment of Antimicrobial Resistance, 2001). It was estimated that more than 50% of antibiotics worldwide are purchased privately without prescriptions from street vendors in the informal sector (Cars & Nordberg,
2005). The practice is often associated with shorter courses of treatment than
is standard, with inappropriate choices of drugs and dosage, and with masking
of the underlying infectious process. All these factors are likely to cause treatment failure and are consequential for antibiotic resistance (Morgan et al., 2011).
A community-based study in Thailand found that bacterial resistance, including penicillin-resistant and erythromycin-resistant *Streptococcus pneumoniae*
was significantly associated with increasing non-prescription use of antibiotics
(Apisarnthanarak & Mundy, 2008).

While this practice is found across the world, it is much more common in developing countries, where sales of antibiotics are less strictly regulated and policies
are ineffectively enforced. The prevalence of non-prescribed use of antibiotics is
less than 1% on average in northern Europe, but it accounts for 19–100% of antibiotic use in areas outside North Europe and North America (Grigoryan et al., 2006,
2010; Morgan et al., 2011). In Asian developing countries, households routinely
stocked antibiotics: 55% of Vietnamese families have antibiotics at home (Okumura et al., 2002), and 42% of the Mongolian caregivers reported having used
non-prescribed antibiotics to treat symptoms in their child during the previous six
months (Togoobaatar et al., 2010).

The practice of self-medication with antibiotics is not rare in China. Although
the Chinese State Food and Drug Administration has enacted measures to forbid
retail pharmacies from selling antibiotics without a prescription (China Food and
Drug Administration, 2003), antibiotics can still be easily purchased without prescriptions for self-medication use (Jiang et al., 2013; Yu et al., 2013). Retail pharmacies have been important suppliers of antibiotics, accounting for more than 30%
of the total volume of sales of antibiotics a year, and the number is still rising
steadily (Wan et al., 2013).

Despite its known existence, research on the caregiver use of non-prescribed
antibiotics, their predictors, and their impact on caregivers' behavior and attitudes
in medical visits is still limited. Bi et al. (2000) reported that 51% of children had
received parental self-medication of antibiotics, and Yu et al. (2014) reported that
62% of parents had used non-prescribed antibiotics with children before medical
visits; however, these studies were based on small samples from one urban city
and two rural counties respectively. Little is known about the prevalence of this
practice across rural and urban areas at varying levels of economic, political, and
cultural development.

Moreover, despite a large body of Western literature on patient desires as an
important contributor to antibiotic overprescription, the effect of caregiver desires
for antibiotic prescriptions in the Chinese respiratory tract infection (RTI) clinical context remains unknown. Research from the UK and the US has shown that
caregiver desires and doctors' perceptions of parental expectations for antibiotics
can significantly increase the likelihood of doctors' overprescription of antibiotics
(Macfarlane et al., 1997; Mangione-Smith et al., 2001; Stivers et al., 2003), and

patient desires were cited by doctors as the most common reason for overprescribing (Elwyn et al., 1999; Epstein et al., 1984; Linder & Singer, 2003). It is, thus, plausible that overprescription of antibiotics and, in particular, antibiotic IV infusions are at least partially due to caregivers' desires for antibiotics in the Chinese pediatric context.

In addition, since self-medication with non-prescribed antibiotics has been a less significant issue for most of the middle-to-high-income countries in Western societies (Grigoryan et al., 2006, 2007, 2008, 2010), its influence on caregivers' health-seeking attitudes such as desires for prescriptions in the visit and, further, on doctors' prescribing decisions has largely remained uninvestigated to this date. Given the prevalence of use of non-prescribed oral antibiotics among caregivers before medical visits and the high prescription rates of IV antibiotic infusions in China, I hypothesize that there is a causal relationship between caregiver use of non-prescribed antibiotics before medical visits, their desires for antibiotic IV infusions in the visit, and doctors' prescriptions of antibiotic prescriptions in the visit.

Furthermore, to identify the predictors of caregivers' use of non-prescribed antibiotics, many studies have found child age as a significant factor (Bi et al., 2000; Yu et al., 2014); other work was mostly concerned with caregivers' knowledge and attitude toward antibiotic use and concluded that low level of knowledge by caregivers of antibiotic use was associated with self-medication (Lv et al., 2014; Yu et al., 2014). However, understanding is lacking with respect to what kinds of caregivers are more prone to these behaviors, that is, their sociodemographic characteristics and their views toward their child's health conditions. The same is true with our understanding of the predictors of caregivers' desires for antibiotic prescriptions and their desires for IV antibiotic prescriptions.

The objective of this study is to estimate the following: (1) the prevalence of non-prescribed antibiotic use by caregivers before medical visits, (2) caregivers' desire for medical services or prescriptions during the visits, and (3) the effect of caregiver desire for antibiotics on prescriptions they receive during the visits. Additionally, the study will identify factors that predict caregivers' pre-visit use of non-prescribed antibiotics and their desire for antibiotic prescriptions. The findings of the study will provide empirical evidence regarding the demand-side factors that contribute to the overprescription of antibiotics, which have been absent from the current research landscape.

Study design

A cross-sectional survey was conducted in China between October and November of 2013. A purposive sampling strategy was used to estimate the prevalence of self-medication, primarily based on a classification of residence. Respondents were recruited from tier 1, tier 2, and tier 3 cities and tier 4 rural districts in China. Tier 1 cities are large, densely populated urban cities with greater economic, cultural, political, and educational resources. Tier 2 cities are generally made up of provincial capitals, subprovincial cities, and other developed cities with cultural and economic influence. Tier 3 cities are mostly made up of open coastal cities, high-income cities, and cities with increasing economic development. Tier 4 districts include townships and villages in rural areas. The data included 34 sites in 21 provinces across the country. Questionnaires were distributed through kindergartens and primary schools to caregivers of children between 3 and 10 years of age. A total of 3,400 questionnaires were distributed, and 3,343 were returned; 3,056 were considered valid (more than 60% of questions answered) and included for data analysis.

Survey instrument

The survey was a self-administered 13-item questionnaire pertaining to children's most recent medical visits to a doctor for cold-like symptoms (a term used in the survey as a vernacular equivalent to ARTI). The survey addressed three main aspects of antibiotic use: (1) caregiver use of non-prescribed antibiotics for the child before their most recent medical visit; (2) doctors' prescribing antibiotics at the visit; (3) visit-related characteristics, such as type of visit (new acute problem vs. follow-up), symptoms at the visit, and services that caregivers requested at the visit. Sociodemographic information on respondents and children was also collected, including age, gender, educational attainment, and monthly household income. The questionnaire was pretested and revised based on a pilot study to improve its accessibility and increase participants' consistency in understanding the questions.

Statistical analysis

Data were entered into EpiData (version 3.1.0) and analyzed with R (version 0.99.467). Descriptive analyses were conducted to obtain an overview of the sociodemographic characteristics of the respondents. Continuous variables such as caregiver's age and child's age are reported with means and standard deviations. Categorical variables such as respondent's gender, educational attainment, household monthly income, and place of residence are described with frequencies and percentages.

Logistic regression was used to identify the sociodemographic determinants of the self-mediation practice. The dependent variable was whether the caregiver reported having used non-prescribed antibiotics before the visit, and the explanatory variables were sociodemographic variables that were included in series models stepwise. These models were then compared based on goodness-of-fit estimates. Odds ratios are reported to describe the effect parameters of the final model. The association between doctors' prescribing of antibiotics and self-medication before the medical visit was tested using the chi-square test of independence.

Sociodemographic characteristics of study participants

The average age of caregivers was 35 years (SD ± 6.7), and the average of children was 7 years (SD ± 1.9). Sixty-seven percent of the respondents were female. A majority of caregivers (78%) were from urban areas (tier 1–3), among which a greater proportion lived in less-urban tier 3 cities (35%), and roughly equal proportions lived in tier 1 and tier 2 cities (22% and 21%, respectively); 22% lived in tier 4 rural areas. Most caregivers reported an education level lower than a college degree, with 31% reporting less than high school, 46% high school or an associate degree, and the remaining 23% a bachelor's degree or above. Nearly half of the respondents reported having a monthly household income lower than RMB 4,000 (USD $615); only 14% of respondents reported having a monthly income higher than RMB 8,000 (USD $1,230). Detailed information is shown in Table 3.1 and Table 3.2.

Clinical characteristics of medical visits

Table 3.3 shows characteristics related to participants' most recent medical visits for children's ARTI symptoms in the past six months. Almost three-quarters of the respondents indicated that their last visit to a doctor was about a new acute problem, and the rest were following up on a previous visit.

On average, each participant reported two symptoms as their reason for the visit. The three most common symptoms were cough, runny nose, and fever, followed by sore throat, loss of appetite, stomachache, vomiting, and shortness of breath. These symptoms are consistent with data about symptom presentation of children in the US and Europe, suggesting that Chinese children are not sicker than North American and European children being seen for ARTIs (DeMuri et al., 2016).

Table 3.1 Sociodemographic characteristics of study respondents

Variable	Mean	SD
Child age	7	1.8
Caregiver age	35	6.7

Table 3.2 Sociodemographic characteristics of caregivers

Variable	Frequency	Percentage
Gender		
Female	1,959	67%
Male	986	33%
Education		
Middle school or less	908	31%
High school or associate degree	1,376	46%
Bachelor's degree or above	678	23%
Residence		
Tier 1	659	22%
Tier 2	652	21%
Tier 3	1,078	35%
Tier 4 (rural)	667	22%

Table 3.3 Clinical characteristics of medical visits

	Frequency	Percentage
Visit type		
Acute	2,067	68%
Follow-up	989	32%
Symptom		
Cough	1,551	51%
Runny nose	1,501	49%
Fever	1,022	33%
Sore throat	865	28%
Bad appetite	652	21%
Stomachache	419	14%
Vomiting	230	8%
Wheezing	123	4%
Other symptoms	63	2%
	Mean	**SD**
Number of symptoms	2	1.2

Table 3.4 Medicine used before medical visit (N=3,020)

Medicine	Frequency	Percentage
Antibiotics	1,161	38%
Non-antibiotics	1,085	36%
None	774	26%
Total	**3,020**	**100%**

Findings

Pre-visit self-medication and use of non-prescribed antibiotics

Table 3.4 shows that a large proportion of caregivers (74%) reported that they had administered medication to their child before visiting a doctor. The medications included non-prescribed antibiotics and Chinese patent anti-inflammatory medicine as well as symptomatic medicine, such as an antipyretic or cough syrup. Among caregivers who administered medication to children, more than half (52%) reported giving non-prescribed antibiotics, accounting for 38% of the total respondents.

This finding shows that the prevalence of pre-visit use of non-prescribed antibiotics is very high among Chinese caregivers and their children across the country. Compared to countries where the sale of antibiotics is strictly regulated, the prevalence is extremely high (38% in China vs. 1% in Europe); the prevalence is also high compared to African countries – 8% in Tanzania (Elfving et al., 2016). Even in Asian countries, where the use of non-prescribed antibiotics has been found to be widespread, the prevalence is also considered to be at the higher end – 5% in Thailand and Myanmar (Althaus et al., 2020), 42% in Mongolia (Togoobaatar et al., 2010). As China is the largest manufacturer and the second largest consumer of antibiotics in the world (Boeckel et al., 2014), the problem of irrational use of non-prescribed antibiotics in the community setting is concerning.

Although there have been national regulations and policies restricting the sale of antibiotics to prescription only, these regulations have not been strictly and effectively enforced. Antibiotics can be easily purchased without prescriptions at retail pharmacies and through online drug stores. As discussed earlier, self-medication with non-prescribed antibiotics contributes to rising levels of bacterial resistance, and the high prevalence of this practice in China means that the threat to public health is particularly pronounced, with increased contact and exchange both domestically and globally.

Desires for antibiotics and IV infusions in medical visit

A total of 74% (n=2,224) of the respondents reported having desires of some kind when they brought their child to visit doctors. Among them, the most common four types of desires are unrelated to medications, including informing about diagnosis (51%), informing about causes of illness (52%), informing about management method of the child's symptoms (51%), and having physical exams by the doctor (51%) (see Table 3.5).

Among those who reported a desire for some kind of prescription from the doctor, the three most common types of prescriptions were oral Chinese anti-inflammatory

Table 3.5 Caregiver desire in medical visit (N=3,004*)

Reported desire[†]	Frequency	Percentage
Informing about diagnosis	1,598	53%
Informing about cause of illness	1,573	52%
Informing about management methods	1,524	51%
Conducting physical exam	1,523	51%
No particular desires/Following doctors' recommendations	780	26%
Chinese anti-inflammatory oral medicine	509	17%
Antibiotic IV infusions	447	15%
Antibiotic oral medicine	400	13%
Non-antibiotic oral medicine	276	9%
Non-antibiotic IV infusions	57	2%
Other	22	1%
	Mean	**SD**
Number of reported desires	2.9	1.63

* Missing data were deleted listwise.
† Caregivers could check any number of these items in the survey.

medicine (23%), antibiotic IV infusions (20%), and antibiotic oral medicine (18%); in contrast, only 12% of them reported desires for non-antibiotic oral medicine (excluding the anti-inflammatory medicine). This indicates that the caregivers most favor antibiotic prescriptions; particularly, between the two modalities of antibiotic prescriptions, antibiotic IV infusions are preferred over oral medicine.

Prescriptions received in medical visit

Prescriptions that patients and caregivers received at visits were investigated in the survey. Table 3.6 shows that 70% of the respondents reported that they had received antibiotic prescriptions from their doctors; among them, 43% of them received antibiotic IV infusions.

Considering Europe and the US, where it is unlikely that children would receive IV antibiotics at such visits, the proportion of children receiving IV antibiotics in China is astonishingly high.

Association between caregiver pre-visit use of non-prescribed antibiotics, desire for antibiotic prescriptions, and prescriptions received

First, caregiver pre-visit use of non-prescribed oral antibiotics was significantly associated with their desire to receive antibiotic IV infusions in medical visits (OR = 1.89, 95% CI: 1.54–2.33). Compared to those who had not used antibiotics before the medical visits, caregivers who had used antibiotics were almost two times more likely to report a desire to receive doctors' antibiotic IV infusion prescriptions.

Second, caregiver pre-visit use of non-prescribed antibiotics was also significantly associated with them receiving antibiotic IV infusion prescriptions in medical visits (X^2 = 32.25, df = 1, p < 0.001). In other words, compared to those who had not used antibiotics before the medical visits, caregivers who used non-prescribed antibiotics were significantly more likely to receive antibiotic IV infusion prescriptions.

Table 3.6 Prescribing decisions in medical visit (N=2,939*)

		Frequency	*Percentage*
Antibiotic		**2,069**	**70%**
	Antibiotic IV infusions	883	43%
	Antibiotic oral medicine	1,186	57%
Non-antibiotic		**870**	**30%**
	Chinese anti-inflammatory medications	512	59%
	Other non-antibiotic medications	358	41%

* Missing data were deleted listwise.

Lastly, to examine the relationship between caregiver desires for antibiotics and prescriptions they received in medical visits, child age, caregiver age, gender, educational attainment, residence place, type of visit, number of symptoms presented at the visit, and number of caregiver self-report desire for the visit were treated as confounding variables. After controlling for these confounding variables, the results of the multiple logistic regressions revealed that caregivers' desires for antibiotic prescriptions were significantly associated with them receiving doctors' antibiotic prescriptions in medical visits (see Table 3.7).

As shown in the table, after controlling for all other variables, caregivers who reported having desire for antibiotic prescriptions were 24.3% more likely to receive antibiotic prescriptions compared to those who did not report such a desire. Caregivers who were younger, with an older child, paying a follow-up visit, presenting more symptoms, and reporting more desires for the visit were significantly more likely to receive antibiotic prescriptions from their doctors than those otherwise. However, caregiver gender, educational attainment, and residence place were not significant.

Predictors of pre-visit use of non-prescribed antibiotics

After adjusting for potential confounding factors using multiple logistic regression and comparing models, it was found that the sociodemographic characteristics of

Table 3.7 Effect of caregiver desire for antibiotics on prescription received in medical visit (N=3,056)

Variable	Odds ratio	95% CI	p-Value	
Caregiver desires for antibiotic prescriptions	1.243	1.191–1.297	<0.0001	***
Visit type	0.949	0.914–0.985	0.006	**
Child age	1.015	1.004–1.026	0.006	**
Caregiver age	0.995	0.992–0.998	0.000	***
Caregiver sex	0.991	0.955–1.029	0.652	
Caregiver education				
Middle school degree or lower	Reference			
High school	0.991	0.946–1.038	0.700	
Association degree	1.043	0.989–1.101	0.121	
College degree	1.014	0.960–1.072	0.609	
Master degree or above	1.000	0.915–1.093	0.998	
Residence place				
Tier 1	Reference			
Tier 2	1.031	0.977–1.089	0.262	
Tier 3	1.011	0.964–1.061	0.646	
Tier 4 (Rural)	0.999	0.946–1.055	0.971	
Number of symptoms	1.041	1.025–1.058	<0.0001	***
Number of desires	1.022	1.010–1.034	<0.001	***

Note: Significant at 0.05 level.

Table 3.8 Predictors of caregiver use of non-prescribed antibiotics before doctor visit

Variable	Odds ratio	95% CI	p-Value
Child age			
Younger	Reference		
Older	1.016	1.005–1.027	0.007 ***
Caregiver age			
Younger	Reference		
Older	0.997	0.994–1.000	0.082
Caregiver sex			
Female	Reference		
Male	1.011	0.972–1.052	0.257
Caregiver education			
Middle school or less	Reference		
High school or associate degree	0.926	0.886–0.968	0.001 ***
Bachelor's degree or above	0.861	0.815–0.908	<0.0001 ***
Residence			
Tier 1	1.119	1.058–1.184	<0.001 ***
Tier 2	1.072	1.020–1.128	0.002 **
Tier 3	1.130	1.006–1.197	<0.001 ***
Tier 4 (rural)	1.045	1.029–1.061	<0.0001 ***

Notes: **Significance at 0.01 level; ***Significance at 0.001 level.

child age, caregiver educational attainment, and place of residence were all significantly associated with the use of non-prescribed antibiotics before medical visits. Table 3.8 shows the effect parameters for the predictors.

Child age was positively associated with caregivers' use of non-prescribed antibiotics before medical visits. Specifically, for each year of increase in a child's age, the likelihood that their caregiver would administer non-prescribed antibiotics increased by 6%. Second, caregiver educational attainment was also a significant predictor. Compared to caregivers with an education level lower than high school, caregivers with a high school education or an associate degree were 26% less likely to administer non-prescribed antibiotics to their child, and those with a bachelor's degree or above were 51% less likely. Third, the caregiver's place of residence was also found to be significantly associated with self-medication. Compared to caregivers living in tier 1 urban districts, those who lived in tier 2 urban districts were 1.7 times more likely to administer non-prescribed antibiotics to their child, followed by rural residents in tier 4 districts, who were 1.6 times more likely, and tier 3 residents, who were 1.3 times more likely.

Predictors of caregivers' desires for antibiotic prescriptions

Table 3.9 shows the effect parameters of the variables that predict caregivers' desires for antibiotic prescriptions. The results revealed that child age, caregiver gender, caregiver educational attainment, residence place, type of visit, number of symptoms presented, number of desires reported, and whether caregiver had used

Table 3.9 Predictors of caregiver desire for antibiotic prescriptions (N=3,056)

Variable	Odds ratio	95% CI	p-Value
Child age	1.021	1.011–1.030	<0.0001***
Caregiver age	1.001	0.998–1.003	0.553
Caregiver sex	0.947	0.917–0.979	0.001 **
Caregiver education			
Middle school degree or lower	Reference		
High school or associate degree	0.951	0.917–0.987	0.008 **
College degree or above	0.891	0.851–0.932	<0.0001***
Residence place			
Tier 1	Reference		
Tier 2	1.042	0.994–1.093	0.080
Tier 3	1.178	1.130–1.229	<0.0001***
Tier 4 (Rural)	1.070	1.017–1.120	0.008 **
Visit type	0.937	0.907–0.969	<0.0001***
Number of symptoms	1.033	1.019–1.047	<0.0001***
Number of desires	1.050	1.040–1.061	<0.0001***
Use of antibiotics before the visit	1.153	1.117–1.191	<0.0001***

Note: **Significance at 0.01 level; ***Significance at 0.001 level.

antibiotics before the visit were all significantly associated with caregivers' desires for antibiotic prescriptions, whereas caregiver age was not.

Specifically, caregivers with older children, who were male, and who had lower educational attainment were more likely to report desires for antibiotic prescriptions; compared to those residing in tier 1 urban areas, caregivers living in tier 2, tier 3 urban areas, and tier 4 rural areas were all more likely to report desires for antibiotics. In addition, caregivers who were paying a follow-up visit, presenting more symptoms, and reporting a higher number of desires were also more likely to report desires for antibiotics. Furthermore, caregivers who had used antibiotics prior to the medical visit were also significantly more likely to report a desire for antibiotic prescriptions.

Interpretations of findings

In this chapter, I examined caregivers' pre-visit use of non-prescribed antibiotics, their desire for antibiotic prescriptions, and the prescriptions they received in medical visits for their child's common cold symptoms. First, more than 70% of the caregivers self-medicate their child's condition with some kind of medicine before the medical visit. Among the medicines used, non-prescribed antibiotics were most common. Second, 28% of caregivers reported having a desire for antibiotic prescriptions in medical visits – IV infusions were preferred over oral ones. Third, the relationships between caregiver pre-visit use of antibiotics, their desire for antibiotic prescriptions, and the prescriptions they received in medical visits were significant. These findings, thus, suggest an association between caregivers' pre-visit medication behavior in the community setting and the prescriptions they receive in the clinical setting.

The impact of pre-visit medication use behavior on doctors' prescribing behavior may come about by two pathways. First, recent research showed that patient use of antibiotics before medical visits was likely to reduce the sensitivity of blood cultures (Vaidya et al., 2020). Thus, the complicated diagnostic test and evaluation results caused by pre-visit use of antibiotics increase the likelihood of overuse and misuse of antibiotics in the clinical setting. Second, pre-visit use of non-prescribed antibiotics is also associated with an increased likelihood that patients will request antibiotic prescriptions at doctor visits. In another study, it was found that when caregivers reported having used non-prescribed antibiotics before visits, they were significantly more likely to report requesting antibiotic prescriptions at doctor visits (Wang, 2017). Such a desire for antibiotic prescriptions, likely communicated through doctor–patient interactions at medical visits, has an impact on doctors' prescribing behavior. Studies in various settings using different approaches have shown that when doctors perceive patient or caregiver pressure in medical interactions, they are significantly more likely to prescribe inappropriately (Linder & Singer, 2003; Mangione-Smith et al., 1999; Stivers, 2007; Wang, 2020; Wang & Liu, 2021).

Furthermore, there is an additional complication related to China's antibiotic overprescription problem. Apart from the overuse and misuse of oral medication, antibiotics are also commonly prescribed in intravenous infusion form (Li et al., 2012; Reynolds & McKee, 2011). As shown in the study's findings, the use of non-prescribed antibiotics is almost a prevailing medical culture among Chinese caregivers when managing children's common cold symptoms. When caregivers take children to doctors' offices, many of them have already used the doctors' frontline treatment, oral antibiotics, which they are not supposed to have access to yet, in practice, are readily available from street-side vendors without a prescription. Their failure to manage their child's condition with non-prescribed oral antibiotics is thus the reason to visit a doctor, and this is frequently translated into doctors being pressured in the medical interaction to prescribe a more effective and 'superior' treatment, IV antibiotics (Reynolds & McKee, 2009). Therefore, not only does pre-visit use of non-prescribed antibiotics increase the likelihood of inappropriate prescribing of antibiotics in the clinical context, but it also exacerbates the antibiotic resistance problem by expanding their misuse.

Identifying predictors of the use of non-prescribed antibiotics is important to develop policies and interventions to reduce the inappropriate use of antibiotics in high-risk population groups. First, it is found that the older age of children is associated with a higher likelihood of caregiver administration of non-prescribed antibiotics. This is in line with findings from previous studies (Togoobaatar et al., 2010; Yu et al., 2014). Similar to the interpretation of the Mongolian study (Togoobaatar et al., 2010), caregivers in China are also likely to be more careful with younger children and, thus, more likely to bring them to medical visits without administering medication beforehand. In addition, caregivers may have accumulated experience in managing minor ailments and will be more likely to treat their children by themselves as the children grow older; only when conditions cannot be managed with self-medication would those caregivers bring their children to medical visits.

Second, the finding that caregiver educational attainment is a significant predictor of self-medication is also related to the earlier finding that a lower level of knowledge of antibiotic use is associated with caregiver medication practices (Yu et al., 2014). Although this study did not directly examine caregivers' knowledge of antibiotic use, their level of education is quite possibly a more fundamental contributor. Caregivers who have higher educational attainment are more likely to have more social and economic resources and access to knowledge about rational antibiotic use and, thus, may also be more cautious about using antibiotics without a prescription for their children. However, they comprise a minority of caregivers in China and most other countries.

Additionally, the findings of this study also highlight the effect of the caregiver's place of residence as a significant factor. Most previous studies investigated self-medication based on samples from a single urban or rural area; therefore, it was not possible to make conclusions about relative risks across different residence classifications. Furthermore, the finding that caregivers in tier 2 urban districts, rather than rural areas, were the most likely to administer non-prescribed antibiotics for their children was surprising. One possible explanation is that, compared to rural districts, the unregulated sale of antibiotics at retail pharmacies is more common in tier 2 urban districts.

Conclusion

The overuse of antibiotics, especially without a prescription, has led to an increase in antibiotic resistance. Although this practice is prevalent in China, few studies have estimated its national prevalence in both urban and rural areas. Additionally, while much research has been conducted on the overprescription of antibiotics in clinical settings, little is known about whether doctors' prescribing behavior is influenced by patient caregivers' use of non-prescribed antibiotics and expectations for antibiotics before medical visits in the community setting. This study adds to the existing literature in this regard.

The findings of the study suggest that enacting effective regulations and enforcing strict policies on restricted access to antibiotics in retail markets are important for reducing the non-prescribed use of antibiotics in the community. This, in turn, can decrease caregivers' irrational demand for antibiotics and the prescription of antibiotics in clinical settings. Programs aimed at reducing the use of non-prescribed antibiotics in the community can prioritize targeting high-risk population groups such as caregivers with school-age children and those with lower educational levels residing in tier 2 urban and rural districts.

Finally, improving patients' health-seeking behavior and attitudes toward antibiotics has the potential to address the problem of overprescription in clinical settings. As shown in Western literature, patients' and caregivers' expectations and health-seeking behaviors, even before the medical visit, significantly influence doctors' prescriptions. These influences can be carried over to the medical visit and conveyed through their interaction with doctors. In the next chapter, I will examine the interactional practices commonly used by patient caregivers to advocate for antibiotics in medical visits.

References

Althaus, T., Thaipadungpanit, J., Greer, R. C., Swe, M. M. M., Dittrich, S., Peerawaranun, P., Smit, P. W., Wangrangsimakul, T., Blacksell, S., Winchell, J. M., Diaz, M. H., Day, N. P. J., Smithuis, F., Turner, P., & Lubell, Y. (2020). Causes of fever in primary care in Southeast Asia and the performance of C-reactive protein in discriminating bacterial from viral pathogens. *International Journal of Infectious Diseases: IJID: Official Publication of the International Society for Infectious Diseases*, *96*, 334–342. https://doi.org/10.1016/j.ijid.2020.05.016

Apisarnthanarak, A., & Mundy, L. M. (2008). Correlation of antibiotic use and antimicrobial resistance in Pratumthani, Thailand, 2000 to 2006. *American Journal of Infection Control*, *36*(9), 681–682. https://doi.org/10.1016/j.ajic.2007.10.022

Bi, P., Tong, S., & Parton, K. A. (2000). Family self-medication and antibiotics abuse for children and juveniles in a Chinese city. *Social Science & Medicine*, *50*(10), 1445–1450.

Boeckel, T. P. V., Gandra, S., Ashok, A., Caudron, Q., Grenfell, B. T., Levin, S. A., & Laxminarayan, R. (2014). Global antibiotic consumption 2000 to 2010: An analysis of national pharmaceutical sales data. *The Lancet Infectious Diseases*, *14*(8), 742–750. https://doi.org/10.1016/S1473-3099(14)70780-7

Cars, O., & Nordberg, P. (2005). Antibiotic resistance – The faceless threat. *International Journal of Risk & Safety in Medicine*, *17*(3,4), 103–110.

CFDA. (2003). *Notice on strengthening the supervision of antibiotic sales in retail pharmacies and promoting rational drug use*. China Food and Drug Administration. http://www.sda.gov.cn/WS01/CL0055/10126.html

DeMuri, G. P., Gern, J. E., Moyer, S. C., Lindstrom, M. J., Lynch, S. V., & Wald, E. R. (2016). Clinical features, virus identification, and sinusitis as a complication of upper respiratory tract illness in children ages 4–7 years. *The Journal of Pediatrics*, *171*, 133–139. e1. https://doi.org/10.1016/j.jpeds.2015.12.034

Elfving, K., Shakely, D., Andersson, M., Baltzell, K., Ali, A. S., Bachelard, M., Falk, K. I., Ljung, A., Msellem, M. I., Omar, R. S., Parola, P., Xu, W., Petzold, M., Trollfors, B., Björkman, A., Lindh, M., & Mårtensson, A. (2016). Acute uncomplicated febrile illness in children aged 2–59 months in Zanzibar – Aetiologies, antibiotic treatment and outcome. *PloS One*, *11*(1), e0146054. https://doi.org/10.1371/journal.pone.0146054

Elwyn, G., Gwyn, R., Edwards, A., & Grol, R. (1999). Is "shared decision-making" feasible in consultations for upper respiratory tract infections? Assessing the influence of antibiotic expectations using discourse analysis. *Health Expectations: An International Journal of Public Participation in Health Care and Health Policy*, *2*(2), 105–117.

Epstein, A. M., Read, J. L., & Winickoff, R. (1984). Physician beliefs, attitudes, and prescribing behavior for anti-inflammatory drugs. *The American Journal of Medicine*, *77*(2), 313–318.

Grigoryan, L., Burgerhof, J. G. M., Degener, J. E., Deschepper, R., Lundborg, C. S., Monnet, D. L., Scicluna, E. A., Birkin, J., Haaijer-Ruskamp, F. M., & Self-Medication with Antibiotics and Resistance (SAR) Consortium. (2008). Determinants of self-medication with antibiotics in Europe: The impact of beliefs, country wealth and the healthcare system. *The Journal of Antimicrobial Chemotherapy*, *61*(5), 1172–1179. https://doi.org/10.1093/jac/dkn054

Grigoryan, L., Burgerhof, J. G. M., Haaijer-Ruskamp, F. M., Degener, J. E., Deschepper, R., Monnet, D. L., Di Matteo, A., Scicluna, E. A., Bara, A.-C., Lundborg, C. S., Birkin, J., & SAR group. (2007). Is self-medication with antibiotics in Europe driven by prescribed use? *The Journal of Antimicrobial Chemotherapy*, *59*(1), 152–156. https://doi.org/10.1093/jac/dkl457

Grigoryan, L., Haaijer-Ruskamp, F. M., Burgerhof, J. G. M., Mechtler, R., Deschepper, R., Tambic-Andrasevic, A., Andrajati, R., Monnet, D. L., Cunney, R., Di Matteo, A., Edelstein, H., Valinteliene, R., Alkerwi, A., Scicluna, E. A., Grzesiowski, P., Bara, A.-C., Tesar, T., Cizman, M., Campos, J., . . . Birkin, J. (2006). Self-medication with antimicrobial drugs in Europe. *Emerging Infectious Diseases*, *12*(3), 452–459. https://doi.org/10.3201/eid1203.050992

Grigoryan, L., Monnet, D. L., Haaijer-Ruskamp, F. M., Bonten, M. J. M., Lundborg, S., & Verheij, T. J. M. (2010). Self-medication with antibiotics in Europe: A case for action. *Current Drug Safety*, *5*(4), 329–332.

Jiang, M., Fang, Y., Chen, W., Yang, S., Liu, J., & Hou, H. (2013). Status quo on prescription antibiotics in retail pharmacies of Shanxi Province. *Zhong Guo Wei Sheng Zheng Ce Yan Jiu*, *6*, 40–45.

Li, Y., Xu, J., Wang, F., Wang, B., Liu, L., Hou, W., Fan, H., Tong, Y., Zhang, J., & Lu, Z. (2012). Overprescribing in China, driven by financial incentives, results in very high use of antibiotics, injections, and corticosteroids. *Health Affairs*, *31*(5), 1075–1082. https://doi.org/10.1377/hlthaff.2010.0965

Linder, J. A., & Singer, D. E. (2003). Desire for antibiotics and antibiotic prescribing for adults with upper respiratory tract infections. *Journal of General Internal Medicine*, *18*(10), 795–801. https://doi.org/10.1046/j.1525-1497.2003.21101.x

Lv, B., Zhou, Z., Xu, G., Yang, D., Wu, L., Shen, Q., Jiang, M., Wang, X., Zhao, G., Yang, S., & Fang, Y. (2014). Knowledge, attitudes and practices concerning self-medication with antibiotics among university students in western China. *Tropical Medicine & International Health*, *19*(7), 769–779. https://doi.org/10.1111/tmi.12322

Macfarlane, J., Holmes, W., Macfarlane, R., & Britten, N. (1997). Influence of patients' expectations on antibiotic management of acute lower respiratory tract illness in general practice: Questionnaire study. *BMJ*, *315*(7117), 1211–1214. https://doi.org/10.1136/bmj.315.7117.1211

Mangione-Smith, R., McGlynn, E. A., Elliott, M. N., Krogstad, P., & Brook, R. H. (1999). The relationship between perceived parental expectations and pediatrician antimicrobial prescribing behavior. *Pediatrics*, *103*(4), 711–718.

Mangione-Smith, R., McGlynn, E. A., Elliott, M. N., McDonald, L., Franz, C. E., & Kravitz, R. L. (2001). Parent expectations for antibiotics, physician-parent communication, and satisfaction. *Archives of Pediatrics & Adolescent Medicine*, *155*(7), 800–806. https://doi.org/10.1001/archpedi.155.7.800

Morgan, D. J., Okeke, I. N., Laxminarayan, R., Perencevich, E. N., & Weisenberg, S. (2011). Non-prescription antimicrobial use worldwide: A systematic review. *The Lancet Infectious Diseases*, *11*(9), 692–701. https://doi.org/10.1016/S1473-3099(11)70054-8

Okumura, J., Wakai, S., & Umenai, T. (2002). Drug utilisation and self-medication in rural communities in Vietnam. *Social Science & Medicine*, *54*(12), 1875–1886. https://doi.org/10.1016/S0277-9536(01)00155-1

Reynolds, L., & McKee, M. (2009). Factors influencing antibiotic prescribing in China: An exploratory analysis. *Health Policy*, *90*(1), 32–36. https://doi.org/10.1016/j.healthpol.2008.09.002

Reynolds, L., & McKee, M. (2011). Serve the people or close the sale? Profit-driven overuse of injections and infusions in China's market-based healthcare system. *The International Journal of Health Planning and Management*, *26*(4), 449–470. https://doi.org/10.1002/hpm.1112

Stivers, T. (2007). *Prescribing under pressure: Physician-parent conversations and antibiotics*. Oxford University Press.

Stivers, T., Mangione-Smith, R., Elliott, M. N., McDonald, L., & Heritage, J. (2003). Why do physicians think parents expect antibiotics? What parents report vs what physicians believe. *The Journal of Family Practice*, *52*(2), 140–148.

Togoobaatar, G., Ikeda, N., Ali, M., Sonomjamts, M., Dashdemberel, S., Mori, R., & Shibuya, K. (2010). Survey of non-prescribed use of antibiotics for children in an urban community in Mongolia. *Bulletin of the World Health Organization*, *88*(12), 930–936. https://doi.org/10.2471/BLT.10.079004

Vaidya, K., Aiemjoy, K., Qamar, F. N., Saha, S. K., Tamrakar, D., Naga, S. R., Saha, S., Hemlock, C., Longley, A. T., Date, K., Bogoch, I. I., Garrett, D. O., Luby, S. P., & Andrews, J. R. (2020). Antibiotic use prior to hospital presentation among individuals with suspected enteric fever in Nepal, Bangladesh, and Pakistan. *Clinical Infectious Diseases: An Official Publication of the Infectious Diseases Society of America*, *71*(suppl_3), S285–S292. https://doi.org/10.1093/cid/ciaa1333

Wan, Q., Zhang, Y., Wang, X., Zhai, T., Wang, C., & Chai, P. (2013). Results and analysis of China national health accounts in 2013. *Zhong Guo Wei Sheng Jing Ji*, *3*(34), 5–8.

Wang, N. C. (2017). *Social determinants of antibiotic prescribing in China* [PhD dissertation, University of California].

Wang, N. C. (2020). Understanding antibiotic overprescribing in China: A conversation analysis approach. *Social Science & Medicine*, *262*, 113251. https://doi.org/10.1016/j.socscimed.2020.113251

Wang, N. C., & Liu, Y. (2021). Going shopping or consulting in medical visits: Caregivers' roles in pediatric antibiotic prescribing in China. *Social Science & Medicine*, 114075. https://doi.org/10.1016/j.socscimed.2021.114075

WHO Global Strategy for Containment of Antimicrobial Resistance (WHO/CDS/DRS/2001.2). (2001). WHO. http://www.who.int/csr/resources/publications/drugresist/WHO_CDS_CSR_DRS_2001_2_EN/en/

Yu, M., Zhao, G., Lundborg, C. S., Zhu, Y., Zhao, Q., & Xu, B. (2014). Knowledge, attitudes, and practices of parents in rural China on the use of antibiotics in children: A cross-sectional study. *BMC Infectious Diseases*, *14*(1), 112. https://doi.org/10.1186/1471-2334-14-112

Yu, M., Zhu, Y.-P., Song, X.-X., Yang, L., Tao, T., Zhao, Q., Xu, B., & Zhao, G.-M. (2013). Insights into residents' behavior of antibiotic purchasing from medicinal sales data of retail pharmacies in rural China. *Fudan University Journal of Medical Sciences*, *40*(3), 253–258. https://doi.org/10.3969/j.issn.1672-8467.2013.03.001

4 Caregivers' role in prescribing decision

Overt advocacy and interactional pressure in medical visits

Introduction

In Chapter 3, I demonstrated that patient caregivers can impact the problem of antibiotic overprescription even before visiting doctors in clinical settings. Caregivers' expectations, which are associated with their pre-visit use of non-prescribed antibiotics, can carry over to medical interactions with doctors and further influence prescribing decisions. In this chapter, I shift our attention from the outside to the inside of the clinical setting, where the prescribing decisions related to antibiotics are actually made between doctors and patient caregivers in and through interaction.

Following the supply-side theory, if doctors were primarily responsible for the antibiotic overprescription problem and patient caregivers had little to no impact, then it would be unlikely to find caregivers communicating their expectations for antibiotic prescriptions to doctors during medical visits. However, research conducted in various cultural and clinical settings has shown that patients or caregivers do communicate their expectations for antibiotics during medical visits. When doctors perceive these expectations, they are significantly more likely to prescribe antibiotics unnecessarily. Considering the previous chapter's finding that patient caregivers' expectations for antibiotics are common and that their expectations are significantly linked to the prescribing decisions. It is thus reasonable to ask: How and how often do patient caregivers communicate their expectations and desires for antibiotics to their doctors in Chinese pediatric primary care? Furthermore, do these communication practices actually influence doctors' prescribing decisions?

In the following, I present findings related to caregivers' interactional practices that they use and are often understood by doctors as advocating for antibiotic prescriptions in medical interaction. Using conversation analysis, I first show how these language practices are enacted qualitatively in naturally occurring medical conversations. I then illustrate their occurrence and distribution in the dataset and quantitatively examine their effects on prescribing decision outcomes. Finally, I will discuss the implications of these findings by comparing them to related research conducted in the United States. These findings offer crucial evidence for the impact of patients or caregivers, which has been missing from the supply-side theory and our overall understanding of the antibiotic overprescription problem.

DOI: 10.4324/9781003243625-4

Background

Research from the US and UK has shown that antibiotic overprescription is associated with patient desires and expectations (Britten & Ukoumunne, 1997; Choi et al., 2012; Linder & Singer, 2003; Macfarlane et al., 1997). Yet, more in-depth research argues that it is doctors' *perceptions* of parental expectations for antibiotic treatment, rather than actual parental expectations, that are associated with physicians' overprescription (Mangione-Smith et al., 1999, 2006).

This stream of research highlights the crucial role of doctor–patient/parent interaction in antibiotic overprescription. Even when parents do not report an expectation for antibiotics, if physicians infer that they are expecting antibiotics, they are significantly more likely to prescribe inappropriately (Mangione-Smith et al., 1999). Therefore, antibiotic overprescription can be interactionally generated (Britten, 2001; Mangione-Smith et al., 2015; Stivers, 2002a, 2005, 2006, 2007; Stivers et al., 2003a), independent of physicians' professional judgments of patients' medical conditions.

Following this line of research, I examine patient caregivers' influence on antibiotic overprescribing by looking at caregivers' advocating actions in this chapter. At its core, the advocating actions can be understood as recruitment-like actions (Drew & Couper-Kuhlen, 2014; Kendrick & Drew, 2016); that is, by producing such actions, the speaker attempts to enlist someone's assistance, typically with respect to an immediate physical need, problem, or wish, and generates implications of need, of obligation, of imposition, and of constraint (Drew & Couper-Kuhlen, 2014). I first review existing findings regarding (1) requesting as a social action more generally and (2) advocating actions for antibiotic treatment in medical interaction.

Requesting as a delicate action in social interaction

Requesting is one of the most basic and ubiquitous activities in social interaction. Its significance as a social action is reviewed by Drew and Couper-Kuhlen (2014) and can be summarized as having three components. First, we do request very often in daily life – whoever we are and wherever we live, whatever language we speak, whatever work we do, whatever our 'position' in society. Second, requesting lies at the very heart of cooperation and collaboration in our social lives and has a particular significance for our interactions, relationships, and associations with one another – through requesting, we seek the help of others in doing or managing things that we could not do, or could not so easily do, or would prefer not to do by ourselves (Drew & Couper-Kuhlen, 2014; Heritage, 2016; Rossi, 2015). Third, requesting is a delicate matter – when we make requests, we inherently, but usually implicitly, convey that we need something; we expose ourselves to be seen as wanting in some fashion. Moreover, we place some kind of *obligation* on the requestee, one that might require a degree of *imposition* or even sacrifice, some risks to the requester of being turned down or acquiring a reciprocal obligation. As a social action, requesting, thus, carries with it implications of need, of obligation, of imposition, and of constraint and is a core feature of the management of social cohesion and social solidarity in social interaction (Drew & Couper-Kuhlen, 2014, p. 2).

In general, studies of requesting have been concerned with how to map actions onto linguistic expressions (Drew & Couper-Kuhlen, 2014), in other words, the selection of requesting forms and the principles behind people's selections (Rossi, 2015). Despite the large body of literature on this research inquiry, it has mostly been approached from perspectives in psychology (Ervin-Tripp, 1981), language philosophy, and pragmatics – *speech act theory, politeness theory* (Brown & Levinson, 1987). Until recently, researchers on conversation and talk-in-interaction have focused on requesting as a social action. Two central issues being discussed are (1) in what context do speakers design requests in which ways and (2) how does a recipient come to understand a particular linguistic form as implementing a request? (Drew & Couper-Kuhlen, 2014, p. 13). Drew and Couper-Kuhlen (2014) further stated that the most prominent principles to emerge from the discussion in the current literature as relevant for the use of a specific request form include (1) sequential environment, (2) entitlement, and (3) contingency.

Sequential environment is concerned with speakers' understanding of what is going on in the current sequence and/or what has gone on in a prior sequence or sequences. For example, Wootton (1997) analyzed the requesting behavior of a young English-speaking child and found that the child's selection of request forms was sensitive to, and reflexively indicative of, understandings of the interactional context, for example, whether the request was projectably out of line with what the recipient appeared to be envisaging. Similarly, Rossi (2012) identified a functional distinction between imperative and interrogative constructions of requests based on a corpus of naturally occurring Italian interactions – the imperative format was selected to implement 'bilateral requests' (in which the requested actions are integral to an already established joint project between the requester and recipient); whereas the interrogative format was a vehicle for 'unilateral requests' (in which the requested actions seek to enlist help in new, self-contained projects that are launched in the interest of the speaker as an individual).

Entitlement (Curl & Drew, 2008) is concerned with speakers' understanding of whether they have a right to request a particular object or course of action. For instance, Lindström (2005) found that speakers' selection of two requesting forms (i.e., imperatives and interrogatives) depended on their understanding of whether they were entitled to make the request in the context of the Swedish home help services for senior citizens – imperative constructions displayed the requesters' entitlement; whereas the interrogatives indicated otherwise. Similarly, Heinemann (2006), in a similar institutional setting in Denmark, also found requesters using the requesting format *Can't you X?* displayed their entitlement to make the request as compared to the use of the other form *Will you X?*

Contingency is concerned with speakers' awareness or orientation to factors that could compromise the grantability of a request (Drew & Couper-Kuhlen, 2014). Curl and Drew (2008) found that in addition to entitlement, speakers' use of requesting forms (e.g., *Can/could you . . .?* and *I wonder if . . .?*) was also affected by contingency. Specifically, the form *I wonder if . . .?* usually prefaces the requested action that is construed as something that is only possibly an option, due to factors that cannot be anticipated in advance – 'high contingency' requests; whereas the modal construction *Can/Could you . . .?* displays speakers' orientation to fewer contingencies that might affect the grantability of the request – 'low contingency' requests.

In this study, I identify the actions that caregivers use to advocate for antibiotic prescriptions based on the theoretical conceptualization outlined in the existing research. Through using different action designs, caregivers display their orientation toward advocating actions as delicate, if not socially dispreferred, in social encounters. However, the relatively high frequency of their use indicates that patient caregivers actively participate in the decision-making process related to prescribing antibiotics. Next, I briefly review the findings on caregivers' advocating actions in the context of medical consultations and, particularly, Stivers' (2000, 2002a, 2002b, 2005, 2006, 2007) series of research papers on parents' advocating actions for antibiotic treatment in American pediatric acute visits.

Advocating actions in antibiotic prescribing interaction

It is observed that to advocate for antibiotic treatment, American parents primarily rely on covert interactional actions to communicate their desire for or expectation of antibiotic prescriptions in pediatric encounters. These covert advocating actions include *candidate diagnosis*, *diagnosis resistance*, and *passive treatment resistance*. These behaviors have all been shown to be treated by clinicians as a form of pressure for antibiotic prescribing through qualitative analysis.

Offering a candidate diagnosis is one of the two main ways that parents present their child's problems. Stivers (2002b) argues that when the child's problem is presented with a candidate diagnosis, parents are treated as having adopted the stance that they are seeking confirmation of their diagnosis and seeking treatment for the illness condition; whereas when the child's problem is presented with a symptoms-only description, parents are treated as primarily seeking a medical evaluation of the child. Compared to symptoms-only problem presentations, candidate diagnoses were much less frequent – 26% in pediatric encounters; however, when they are used, they are overwhelmingly used to hypothesize bacterial diagnoses, for which antibiotics are a relevant treatment (Stivers, 2007). Although candidate diagnoses do not overtly ask for antibiotics, they constitute a resource through which parents shape physicians' views of the problem and thus influence the treatment decision early in the consultation. Moreover, statistical evidence has revealed that when caregivers used a candidate diagnosis, physicians were five times more likely to perceive caregivers as expecting antibiotic prescriptions (Mangione-Smith et al., 2015; Stivers et al., 2003b).

Mentioning additional symptoms and *mentioning possible diagnoses* are two interactional resources through which parents influence physicians' views of the patient's condition in response to history-taking questions and thus can effectively negotiate treatment decisions (Stivers, 2007). First, *mentioning additional problematic symptoms* works to steer physicians away from a no-problem diagnosis by (1) pushing the physicians toward an alternative diagnostic path by introducing a new dimension of the illness and (2) inviting the physicians' pursuit and sequence expansion that would move the trajectory in a different direction. Second, *mentioning alternative possible diagnoses* is typically used when the physicians' history-taking questions involve or implicate a 'no-problem' answer. By proposing alternative diagnoses, parents work to push the physicians toward a conceptualization of the illness that is at odds with the prior line of questioning. The two covert pressuring practices are not frequently used in the American dataset – 12% and 9%, respectively; however, physicians consistently treat them as indexing a desire for antibiotics (Stivers, 2000, 2007).

Diagnosis resistance generally involves calling into question or disaffiliating with the physician's diagnostic evaluation and thus obstructing the progress of the visit to the next activity – treatment recommendation (Stivers, 2007). It is often accomplished with three sorts of sequence-initiating actions: "newsmarks" (Heritage, 1984; Jefferson, 1981), 'questions about symptoms,' and 'questions about the diagnosis.' Specifically, "newsmarks" (*e.g., Really?* and *It is?*) represent the least strong way of resisting, as they merely seek physicians' reconfirmation and thus promote further informing. 'Questioning an examination finding' is a stronger way of resisting, as it explicitly identifies a problem area of the diagnosis and thus projects a challenge to the physician's professional authority; 'questioning about the diagnosis' is the strongest way of resisting because it questions physicians' medical evaluation of the child's condition – a domain over which the physician is normally treated as having sole responsibility and epistemic ownership (Heath, 1992; Peräkylä, 2006). Resistance to diagnosis is comparatively rare – 17% of the dataset (Stivers, 2007); if it occurs, it has to be explicit because doctors generally do not orient to the need for affirmation of their diagnoses by patients (Stivers et al., 2017). Moreover, as Peräkylä (2006) observes, when diagnosis resistance is produced, it is produced in a "cautious manner," and speakers orient to the doctor's authority in the medical domain.

Treatment resistance is another parent resource to negotiate antibiotic treatment in the treatment stage (Stivers, 2005, 2007). The other covert practices reviewed previously are not directly linked to treatment; however, treatment resistance can directly affect the treatment decision by turning the decision into an explicit negotiation. Specifically, since parents and physicians orient to treatment recommendations as proposals that normatively require parent acceptance, a parent withholding of acceptance of a treatment recommendation is treated as a resisting action – "passive treatment resistance" (Heritage & Sefi, 1992), and if physicians do not alter their treatment recommendation in the face of passive treatment resistance, parents routinely shift to "active treatment resistance," which involves actions that challenge physicians' treatment recommendations (e.g., an alternative treatment proposal) (Stivers, 2005) – active treatment resistance occurs in 19% of the American dataset (Stivers, 2007).

In sum, these covert advocating actions are the primary resources that American parents rely on to communicate their desire for and expectations of antibiotic prescriptions. Apart from the aforementioned covert advocating actions for antibiotic prescriptions, Stivers (2002a) also identified four types of overt actions that American parents very infrequently use to advocate for antibiotics, including (1) *direct requests for antibiotic treatment*, (2) *statements of desire for antibiotic treatment,* (3) *inquiries about antibiotic treatment*, and (4) *mentions of past experience with antibiotic treatment*. These overt advocating actions will be described and discussed in greater detail in the following section where I show that Chinese caregivers are deploying very similar resources, but much more frequently, to advocate for antibiotic treatment in their encounters.

Data and analytical procedures

Based on the naturally occurring medical conversation dataset that I collected for the study, I used mixed methods to examine caregivers' interactional practice advocating for antibiotics (see Appendix 1 for details of the data and methods). First, by using the conversation analysis (CA) analytical approach, I analyzed the decision-making process of antibiotic treatment between doctors and caregivers and identified the language practices that caregivers use to advocate for antibiotic prescriptions. Based on the CA findings, I then examine the bivariate relationship between the identified actions and prescribing outcomes of the medical encounters with quantitative analysis.

Findings

Caregiver overt advocacy for antibiotic treatment

Four types of overt advocating actions are identified, namely, (1) evaluations of treatment effectiveness, (2) inquiries about antibiotic treatment, (3) statements of desire for antibiotic treatment, and (4) explicit requests for antibiotic treatment. These four types of social actions differ in the degree of overtness and caregiver imposition on doctors' responsive actions; however, they all display a high level of agency of the caregivers in the social encounter with their doctors.

Explicit requests for antibiotic treatment

Explicit requests are the most overt form of social action that caregivers use to advocate for antibiotic treatment. By producing an explicit request for antibiotic treatment, the caregivers not only display a high level of agency participating in the treatment decision-making regarding their children's health condition but also a high degree of entitlement in affecting the prescribing outcome. Although rarely seen in the American pediatric context, it is argued that explicit requests constitute the most direct form of overt pressure for doctors (Stivers, 2002a), as they both assert a parent's preference for antibiotics and obligate the doctor to respond to the requests. The following excerpt illustrates an example of explicit request in the Chinese pediatric context (see Excerpt 4.1).

In this example, the child is brought in for a coughing condition. Prior to the data shown in the excerpt, the patient has taken a blood test and finds that there is some indication of bacterial infection, yet the condition is not severe. The doctor recommends treating the child with oral medication, which the grandmother agrees with. The two parties then proceed to decide what specific kind of oral medicine to use for the patient. Two non-antibiotic medicines are recommended to the patient, including a Chinese anti-inflammatory medicine (*Yuxingcao*) and an antipyretic medicine. The grandmother minimally acknowledges it, and the doctor begins to wrap up the treatment recommendation stage and get ready to move forward to the next stage of the medical encounter (line 1).

However, this attempt to move forward is resisted by the grandmother, issuing a confirmation-seeking of the doctor's prescription plan (line 2). In line 3, the doctor provides an explicit confirmation, along with a further explication of the prescription plan (lines 4-5). In response to this, the grandmother brings up the child's fever symptoms, again resisting the trajectory of the consultation toward the next stage (line 6). Although it can be argued that the grandmother's offer of the symptom description in this environment implies a need for additional medical assistance (e.g., treatment), it is not explicitly stated. In response, the doctor makes a suggestion for the patient to drink enough fluid (lines 7 and 9). In this environment, the grandmother makes an explicit request for antibiotic prescriptions (line 10).

Excerpt 4.1 An example of explicit request for antibiotics

D: Doctor
GM: Grandmother

1	D:	好	吧?	就	行了	哎,	就	行了.		
		OK	ba	jiu	xingle	ai	jiu	xingle		
		OK	PRT	just	fine	PRT	just	fine		
		"OK? Then that's fine. That's fine."								
2	GM:	那个	就	行	啦?					
		na-ge	jiu	xing	la					
		that	just	fine	PRT					
		"It'll be fine with just that?"								
3	D:	哎	哎	哎.	我	给	你-			
		ai	ai	ai	wo	gei	ni			
		yeah	yeah	yeah	I	give	you			
		"Yeah, yeah, yeah. I'll give you–"								
4		这	次	不	一定	配	了.			
		zhe	ci	bu	yiding	pei	le			
		this	time	not	definitely	prescribe	PT			
		"Then this time it's not necessary to prescribe it."								
5		你	鱼腥草	蒲地蓝	吃	一个	就	可以	了.	
		ni	Yuxingcao	Pudilan	chi	yi-ge	jiu	keyi	le	
		you	Yuxingcao	Pudilan	take	one	just	fine	PT	
		"Yuxingcao or Pudilan, you can just take one of them."								
6	GM:	他-	他	有点	发烧	的	呀,			
			ta	ta	youdian	fashao	de	ya		

(Continued)

Excerpt 4.1 (Continued)

		he	he	a little	fever	PT	PRT		
		"He- he has a little fever."							

7	D:	低	烧	低	烧	多	喝	水	哦.
		di	shao	di	shao	duo	he	shui	o
		low	fever	low	fever	more	drink	water	PRT
		"Low fever, low fever. Drink more water, OK?"							

8	GM:	哦:,	多	喝	水.
		o	duo	he	shui
		OK	more	drink	water
		"OK, drink more water."			

9	D:	哎	哎.
		ai	ai
		yeah	yeah
		"Yeah, yeah."	

10->	GM:	再	配	点	消炎	药.
		zai	pei	dian	xiaoyan	yao
		also	prescribe	some	antibiotic	medicine
		"Also prescribe some antibiotic medicine."				

11	D:	头孢	了	哦,	消炎	药.
		toubao	le	o	xiaoyan	yao
		Cephalo	ASP	PRT	antibiotic	medicine
		"(Then that's) Cephalo, OK? Antibiotic medicine."				

12	GM:	哦:.
		o
		OK
		"OK."

13	D:	你	要	开	点	那个-	那个,
		ni	yao	kai	dian	na-ge	na-ge
		you	want	prescribe	some	that	that
		"You want to be prescribed some of that- that,"					

14		要么	开	一盒	头孢	给	你	吧.
		yao-me	kai	yi-he	tou-bao	gei	ni	ba
		or	prescribe	one-pack	Cephalo	to	you	PRT
		"Or (I'll) prescribe one pack of Cephalo to you, OK?"						

15		实在	说	不	行
		shi-zai	shuo	bu	xing
		indeed	say	not	work
		"If it really doesn't work,"			

16		你	就	吃	两	天	好	吧?
		ni	jiu	chi	liang	tian	hao	ba
		you	just	take	two	day	ok	PRT
		"then you take Cephalo for two days, OK?"						

17	GM:	好.
		hao
		good
		'OK.'

PRT: Particle

Since the doctor has previously stated that the non-antibiotic prescription is already enough for the patient and that the fever symptom can be properly addressed by drinking more fluid, the grandmother's explicit request for an antibiotic prescription thus directly counters the doctor's stance, putting the doctor under a substantial amount of pressure to respond and prescribe.

The doctor also displays herself as under pressure in the face of such overt advocacy. In response to the request, the doctor first seeks the grandmother's confirmation that she is asking for Western antibiotic medicine (*Cephalo*) in line 11. The doctor's action is considered as resisting the request because, rather than granting the antibiotic immediately, she provides the grandmother with another opportunity to retreat from the request. The vernacular name (*Xiaoyan yao*) can be understood as either Western antibiotics or Chinese anti-inflammatory medicine. Although the doctor displays her understanding that the grandmother is requesting antibiotics, she defers the point of giving out the antibiotic prescription. In addition, although the doctor concedes to prescribe Western antibiotics to the patient, her recommendation is, nonetheless, designed as a contingency plan (Mangione-Smith et al., 2001) – *if it really doesn't work, you could take Cephalo for two days, ok?* This, thus, leaves the discretion of using the antibiotic prescription to the grandmother yet, at the same time, reclaims some degree of medical authority by giving instructions.

Statement of desire for antibiotic treatment

Caregivers sometimes state their desire to have, or not to have, some particular type of treatment. Different from explicit requests, statements of desire do not obligate doctors to respond explicitly as to whether the desired prescription will be provided; nevertheless, they still constitute a rather overt form of pressure for doctors to prescribe. In the Chinese pediatric context, it is observed that the statements of desire for antibiotic treatment can usually take two forms: (1) positive-format statements – desire for antibiotic treatment and (2) negative-format statements – desire not to have non-antibiotic treatment. Between the two forms of statements, the positive-format statements are more overt, as they explicitly nominate the treatment being advocated for whereas the negative-format statements are less overt, as they imply a preferred treatment by ruling out a dispreferred one through the implementation of a scalar implicature.

Positive-format statement of desire for antibiotic treatment

Excerpt 4.2 illustrates an example of a caregiver's positive-format statement, which directly nominates the desired treatment. In this example, the child is visiting for a stomachache and headache. Prior to the visit, the patient had coughed for a few days, and the caregiver had given her oral antibiotics and cough syrup for five days already. The doctor suggests the patient take a blood test, and the grandmother accepts the test recommendation (lines 1 to 7). Just before the grandmother and the patient leave to take the blood test, the grandmother states her desire for antibiotic IV treatment (lines 9-12).

Excerpt 4.2 An example of positive-format statement of desire for antibiotics

D: Doctor
GM: Grandmother
P: Patient

1	D:	查		个		指头	血?			
		cha		ge		zhitou	xue			
		examine		CT		finger	blood			

"Take a finger blood test?"

2		(0.5)

3	GM:	行		呢		行	呢.	这个	要	呢.
		xing		ne		xing	ne	zhe-ge	yao	ne
		Alright		PRT		alright	PRT	this	need	PRT

"Alright, alright. This is needed."

4	P:	指头		血?
		zhitou		xue
		finger		blood

"Finger blood?"

5	D:	对.
		dui
		right

"Right."

6		((5 lines of discussion of patient age omitted))

7	GM:	好,		谢谢		哦.
		hao		xiexie		o
		ok		thanks		PRT

"OK. Thanks."

8		((Patient and caregivers getting ready to leave the room))

9->	GM:	哎,		这个		不能	待	哦.
		ai		zhe-ge		buneng	dai	o
		yeah		this		can't	wait	PTR

"Mmm, this can't wait."

10		一开始		就		要	挂,
		yikaishi		jiu		yao	gua
		beginning		just		need	drip

"(She) has to have an IV drip from the very beginning."

11		像	这		种	小	孩子	哦,
		xiang	zhe		zhong	xiao	haizi	o
		like	this		kind	little	kid	PRT

"With little kids like her,

12		正常	吃		药	都	吃	不	好.
		zhengchang	chi		yao	dou	chi	bu	hao
		normal	take		medicine	all	take	not	well

oral medication normally wouldn't work."

13	D:	上	中班		了	哎?
		shang	zhongban		le	ai
		go	lower kindergarten		ASP	PRT

"(She) is in lower kindergarten?"

(Continued)

Excerpt 4.2 (Continued)

14	GM:	大班.					
		daban					
		upper kindergarten					
		"Upper kindergarten."					
15	D:	大班	应该	好	点	了	哎.
		daban	yinggai	hao	dian	le	ai
		upper kindergarten	should	better	bit	ASP	PRT
		"Upper kindergarten, (she) should be a bit better."					

CT: Count
PRT: Particle
ASP: Aspect marker

As shown in this example, even before the blood test is taken, the grandmother states her desire for antibiotic IV treatment outright. Although the statement of desire for antibiotic IV treatment does not explicitly obligate the doctor to respond, the doctor still responds by contesting the grandmother's premise for her treatment advocacy – the patient is not old enough to get well without taking antibiotic IV treatment, thus resisting the caregiver's pressure for prescribing.

Negative-format statement of desire for antibiotic treatment

Caregivers' negative-format statements of desire explicate their preference against some particular treatment; by scalar implicature, they are understood as advocating for some alternative treatment that is preferred better. For instance, in the context of Chinese pediatrics, a dispreference for oral medication is usually understood as a preference for IV treatment, which is considered to be stronger than oral medication and more advanced. Excerpt 4.3 illustrates an example.

In this example, the child has been coughing for more than a week. The grandmother had used oral antibiotics and cough syrup for the child prior to the visit. After taking a blood test, the result finds no sign of bacterial infection. The doctor here prepares to make a treatment recommendation. Before the actual recommendation is delivered, the doctor first asks about the patient's energy level (line 1). This is followed by a question regarding the patient's treatment history – whether the patient tends to use antibiotic IV treatment for similar conditions (line 3). In juxtaposition with this inquiry about the patient's treatment preference in the past, the doctor offers a recommendation of oral medication for the current condition (line 4). In response to this oral treatment recommendation, the grandfather produces a negative-format statement that the patient does not want oral medication.

Excerpt 4.3 An example of negative-format statement of desire for antibiotics

D: Doctor
GM: Grandmother
GF: Grandfather

1	D:	哎,	精神	现在	还	好.	
		ai	jingshen	xianzai	hai	hao	
		yeah	spirit	now	still	alright	
		"Ah, (his) spirit is alright now."					
2	GM:	哎.					
		ai					
		yeah					
		"Yeah."					
3	D:	你	每	次	都	挂水	啊?
		ni	mei	ci	dou	guashui	a
		you	every	time	all	drip	PRT
		"You have drip every time?"					
4		你	吃	点	药,	怎么样	啊?
		ni	chi	dian	yao	zenmeyanga	
		you	take	some	medication	how	PRT
		How about you take some oral medication?"					
5->	**GF:**	药,	他	不	想	吃	药.
		yao	ta	bu	xiang	chi	yao
		medication	he	not	want	take	medication
		"(Oral) medication, he doesn't want to take oral medication."					
6	GM:	挂水.					
		gua-shui					
		drip					
		"(He) wants to have drip."					
7	D:	挂水	是	啊?			
		guashui	shi	a			
		drip	is	PRT			
		"Drip, is it?"					
8	GM:	挂-	挂水	快	一点.		
		gua	guashui	kuai	yidian		
		drip	drip	fast	a little		
		"Drip, is a little faster."					
9	D:	好	呢,	行	呢.		
		hao	ne	xing	ne		
		OK	PRT	alright	PRT		
		"OK. Alright.					
10		那	就	给	你	挂	吧.
		na	jiu	gei	ni	gua	ba
		then	just	give	you	drip	PRT
		Then (I'll) just put you on drip."					

PRT: Particle

Since the negative-format evaluations rely on scalar implicature for the understanding of the treatment advocacy, a positive-format can be used as an escalation of treatment advocacy following the negative-format desire statement. This can be seen in this example: Following the grandfather's statement of desire against oral medication (line 5), the grandmother states positively a desire for antibiotic IV treatment (line 6). Subsequently, the doctor concedes to offer antibiotic IV treatment (lines 9-10).

Inquiry about antibiotic treatment

Besides explicit requests and statements of desire for antibiotic treatment, another type of social action that caregivers frequently use to advocate for antibiotic treatment is inquiries. By asking about the antibiotic treatment in the consultation, caregivers raise antibiotic treatment for discussion with their doctor, thus indicating an interest or understanding of its relevance. Moreover, the question creates an interactional imperative, which obligates the doctor to produce a type-conforming response regarding whether antibiotic treatment is needed (Raymond, 2003). It is in this sense that inquiries about antibiotic treatment constitute an overt advocating action. Excerpt 4.4 illustrates a case of caregiver inquiry.

In this example, the patient is visiting for a coughing complaint. After a physical examination (line 1), the doctor delivers the diagnosis that the child is catching a cold (line 2). Receiving no uptake from the parent (line 3), the doctor repeats the diagnosis and delivers an oral medication treatment recommendation in conjunction with the diagnosis (lines 4–5). Following the doctor's recommendation of oral treatment, the mother pauses for four seconds (line 6) and produces an inquiry about antibiotic IV treatment – *No drip?* (line 7).

Excerpt 4.4 An example of inquiry about antibiotics

D: Doctor
M: Mother

---

1   ((Doctor examining patient's throat))

2 D: 感冒　了.
      gan- le
        mao
      cold   PRT
      "(He's got) a cold."

3   (1.5)

4 D: 感冒,　有点　气管　　炎症.
      gan- you- qi-guan   yan-zheng
        mao   dian
      cold   a little airway   inflammation
      "(He's got) a cold. A little inflammation in the airway.

5   吃　　点　　药　　　　吧?
      chi   dian   yao   ba
      take some medication PRT

(*Continued*)

Excerpt 4.4 (Continued)

		Take some oral medicine, OK?"							
6		(4.0)							
7>	**M:**	不	挂水	啊?					
		bu	gua-shui	a					
		no	drip	PRT					
		"No drip?"							
8	D:	呃,	挂水	不	需要	吧,	先	吃	点	药.
		e	gua-shui	bu	xuyao	ba	xian	chi	dian	yao
		uh	drip	no	need	PRT	first	take	some	medication
		"Uh, no need for drip. Take some (oral) medication first.

9	能	吃	药	好	就	尽量	吃	药	好.
	neng	chi	yao	hao	jiu	jinliang	chi	yao	hao
	can	take	medication	well	then	best	take	medication	well
	(If he) can get well with oral medication, just try the best to take oral medication, OK?"

10	M:	哦,	好.
		o	hao
		okay	OK
		"OK, OK."

PRT: Particle

The inquiry about antibiotic IV treatment, although produced in a position following the doctor's treatment recommendation, nonetheless, initiates a new sequence, making relevant the doctor's explicit answer regarding the need for antibiotic IV treatment for the patient's condition. In addition, the fact that the suggested antibiotic IV treatment directly counters the doctor's proposal for oral medication thus displays a high level of entitlement in participating in the decision-making process in the medical encounter.

The doctor's response (line 8) provides evidence that the mother's inquiry is understood as advocating for treatment rather than mere information seeking. First, the doctor's response is prefaced with *uh,* marking her turn as a dispreferred response to the mother's questions (Kendrick & Torreira, 2015; Pomerantz, 1984). Second, the answer that the antibiotic IV treatment is not necessary is produced with mitigation – the final particle *ba* reduces the assertiveness of the answer, making it a proposal in effect (Li & Thompson, 1981). Third, the doctor's response also changes the topical agenda of the mother's question, as the original question concerns what the doctor is going to do, whereas the doctor's response is designed as an evaluation of the patient's health status, which implies no need for the IV treatment – a transformative answer (Stivers & Hayashi, 2010). Fourth, the re-offering of the oral medication recommendation is made contingent upon the prognosis of the condition, displaying a retreat from the doctor's previous stance. Lastly, the re-offering of the recommendation is accounted for by the doctor with a rationale for the choice of treatment. Together, these features demonstrate that the doctor understands the mother's inquiry not as a question but rather as a social action to advocate for antibiotic IV treatment.

Evaluations of treatment effectiveness

Evaluations of past treatment involve caregivers' assessments of the effectiveness of some particular treatment. The treatment being evaluated can be used for the condition under consultation prior to the visit, or it can be in a more general sense. Similar to statements of desires, the evaluations are usually produced in two formats: (1) positive evaluations and (2) negative evaluations. Positive evaluations imply a preference for a treatment, whereas negative evaluations work less directly by implying a dispreference for treatment and, thus, a preference for an alternative treatment.

Positive evaluations

Excerpt 4.5 illustrates an example of positive evaluation of an antibiotic IV treatment of the caregiver. In this example, the patient is brought in for a coughing condition. After a physical examination, the doctor diagnoses the patient with tracheitis. Here, the doctor suggests the patient take azithromycin, an oral antibiotic (line 1). The mother resists it, informing the doctor that she has already given the patient oral azithromycin for two days prior to the visit (lines 2 to 6). The discussion regarding the use of non-prescribed oral antibiotics continues through line 7 to line 9; while the doctor is working on medical records (line 10), the caregiver produces a positive evaluation of antibiotic IV treatment at line 11.

Excerpt 4.5 An example of positive evaluation

D: Doctor
M: Mother

1	D:	我		建议	你	还是	吃-	吃	点	阿奇霉素.		
		wo		jianyi	ni	haishi	chi	chi	dian	Aqimeisu		
		I		suggest	you	still	take	take	some	Azithromycin		
		"I suggest you still take some oral azithromycin."										
2	M:	阿奇霉素-		就是	吃	了	阿奇霉素.					
		Aqimeisu		jiushi	chi	le	Aqimeisu					
		Azithromycin		just	take	ASP	Azithromycin					
		"Azithromycin- oral azithromycin is just what (we) took."										
3	D:	已经		吃	了	啊?	吃	了	几	天	啦?	
		yijing		chi	le	a	chi	le	ji	tian	a	
		already		take	ASP	PRT	take	ASP	how many	CT	PRT	
		"(You've) already taken it? For how many days?"										
4	M:	吃		了	两	天	了.					
		chi		le	liang	tian	le					
		take		ASP	two	CT	ASP					

(Continued)

Excerpt 4.5 (Continued)

		"(We've) been taking it for two days."						

5　D:

吃	了	两	天	啦?
chi	le	liang	tian	la
take	ASP	two	CT	PRT

"For two days?"

6　M:

嗯,	咳	得	狠	呢.
en	ke	de	hen	ne
yeah	cough	ASP	bad	PRT

"Yeah. (He) coughed really bad."

7　D:

你	吃	了	多少	啊?
ni	chi	le	duoshao	a
you	take	ASP	how much	PRT

"How much did you take?"

8　M:

吃	一	颗.
chi	yi	ke
take	one	CT

"One pill (at a time)."

9　D:

哦,	九	岁	要	吃	一	片	半.
o	jiu	sui	yao	chi	yi	pian	ban
Ok	nine	year-old	need	take	one	CT	half

"Ok. A nine-year-old needs to take one and a half."

10　　　((Doctor working on medical records))

11->M:

挂水	来	得	快.
guashui	lai	de	kuai
drip	work	ASP	fast

"Drip works fast."

12　D:

你	要	挂水	啊?
ni	yao	guashui	a
you	want	drip	PRT

"You want drip?"

13　M:

哎.
ai
yeah

"Yeah."

ASP: Aspect marker
PRT: Particle
CT: Count

The mother positively evaluates antibiotic IV treatment and explicates the advantage that it has (over oral medication) – IV treatment takes effect faster (line 11). Note that the evaluation is produced in an environment where the doctor is implying an oral treatment recommendation with an increase in dosage (line 9). Thus, the caregiver's positive evaluation of antibiotic IV treatment is hearable as a resistance to the oral treatment and advocacy for the antibiotic IV treatment. The doctor's response clearly registers such understanding. Following the mother's positive evaluation of antibiotic IV treatment, the doctor seeks the mother's confirmation of her understanding – *You want IV treatment?* (line 12). This is subsequently confirmed by the mother (line 13).

Negative evaluations

Similar to a negative-format statement of desire, negative evaluations are frequently used by caregivers to advocate for a desirable treatment through the implementation of scalar implicature. By evaluating a treatment negatively, the caregiver displays a dispreference for the treatment and, thereby, implies a preference for an alternative treatment. Excerpt 4.6 illustrates an example of a caregiver's negative evaluation of oral medication – an advocacy for antibiotic IV treatment.

In this example, the child is brought in for his fever. The blood test result shows no sign of bacterial infection. Here, the doctor suggests putting the patient on oral medication (line 1). Receiving no uptake from the caregivers, hearable as "passive resistance" (Heritage & Sefi, 1992; Stivers, 2005) to the oral medication recommendation, the doctor pursues the caregivers' acceptance by mentioning again the blood test results (line 3). In overlap with the doctor's pursuit of acceptance, the grandmother produces a negative evaluation of oral treatment at line 4.

Excerpt 4.6 An example of negative evaluation

D: Doctor
GM1: Grandmother 1

1	D:	实际上	啊,	你		这个	还	要	继续 吃 药.
		shijishang	a	ni		zhege	hai	yao	jixu chi yao
		actually	PRT	you		this	still	need	continue take medication
		"Actually, with this (hemogram),							
		you still need to go on taking (oral) medication."							
2		(.)							
3	D:	[你	这个	血象	啊-				
		ni	zhege	xuexiang	a				
		you	this	hemogram	PRT				
		"Your hemogram"							
4->	GM1:	[没的	用	哎,					
		meide	yong	ai					
		no	use	PRT					
		"It won't work."							
5	D:	你	这个	血象	也	不	高	哎,	
		ni	zhege	xuexiang	ye	bu	gao	ai	
		you	this	hemogram	also	not	high	PRT	
		"Your hemogram isn't high."							

PRT: Particle

Here, the grandmother's negative evaluation concerns the effectiveness of the oral medication (likely due to past experience with the treatment for similar conditions). Being produced in an environment where the doctor's recommendation for oral medication is pending acceptance, the grandmother's negative evaluation of the oral medication constitutes an active form of resistance to the doctor's treatment recommendation (Stivers, 2005), and thereby implies advocacy for antibiotic IV treatment, which is considerably more advanced and effective than oral medication (Reynolds & Mckee, 2009). Similar to statements of desire, evaluations constitute one type of social action that does not require any specific type of response from their recipients. Compared to actions such as explicit requests and inquiries about antibiotic treatment, they are a relatively less overt form of advocacy. However, evaluations are a less overt form of advocacy than statements of desire, as the condition is treated as the central topical agenda (Hayano, 2012) rather than the speaker's desires, embodying a lower degree of agency in their turn design. Therefore, in this example, the doctor could have sought the caregiver's confirmation as to whether they want antibiotic IV treatment instead, like in the previous example; however, the doctor mentions the blood test result again, further pursuing the caregiver's acceptance to her original oral treatment recommendation (line 5).

Frequency of the advocating actions

Based on the conversation analytical study of the caregivers' overt advocating actions in Chinese pediatric encounters, I examine the frequency of these overt advocating actions in the dataset. Table 4.1 shows the number of encounters in which each type of action is observed and the percentage of the complete dataset.

In total, caregivers' overt advocating actions are observed in 100 medical encounters, 54% the Chinese dataset (N=187). This percentage is strikingly high, when compared to what is observed in similar settings in the American context. Stivers (2002a) found that these similar social actions were used by the American parents to participate in treatment decisions regarding their children's ARTIs conditions; however, they were observed only 9% of the time in the American pediatric encounters.

In addition, among these four types of overt advocating actions, inquiries about antibiotic treatment are the most frequently observed, in 50 medical encounters; whereas explicit requests for antibiotic treatment are the least frequently observed, in 10 medical encounters. This distributional pattern is found to be similar to that in the American context. In both contexts, despite the fact that various interactional resources exist for the caregivers to choose from to influence the treatment decision outcome, explicit requests for antibiotic treatment are the least frequently used.

Effects of caregiver overt advocacy on antibiotic prescribing outcomes

To test whether caregivers' use of overt treatment advocacy for antibiotics is associated with doctors' prescribing decisions, a chi-square test of independence is used. The caregivers' use of overt treatment advocacy for antibiotics is operated through a binary variable indicating whether any of the four advocating actions is observed in a visit, whereas the doctors' prescribing decisions are operated through three different binary variables, showing (1) whether

Table 4.1 Caregiver overt advocating actions for antibiotic treatment (N=187*)

Action type	Number of visits in which this is observed	Percentage of visits in which this is observed
Evaluations of treatment effectiveness e.g., *Oral medication won't work.*	26	14%
Inquiries about antibiotic treatment e.g., *Does he need any IV drip?*	50	27%
Statements of desire for antibiotic treatment e.g., *He doesn't want to take oral medicine.*	14	7%
Explicit requests for antibiotic treatment e.g., *(Could you) prescribe us some oral antibiotics?*	10	6%
Total number of visits with one or more actions	**100**	**54%**

* *Note:* Total number of acute visits is 187.

Table 4.2 Test statistics for caregiver use of advocating actions and prescribing outcome (N=187)

	No antibiotics	Antibiotics		*X2 (P)*	
Without advocating action	48	28			
With advocating action	39	72			
Total	87	100	187	**13.135 (0.0003)**	***
	No oral antibiotics	**Oral antibiotics**		*X2 (P)*	
Without advocating action	60	74			
With advocating action	27	26			
Total	87	100	187	0.3592 (0.549)	
	No drip antibiotics	**Drip antibiotics**		*X2 (P)*	
Without advocating action	75	54			
With advocating action	12	46			
Total	87	100	187	**21.075 (<0.0001)**	***

Note:**Significance at 0.01 level; ***Significance at 0.001 level.

antibiotics are prescribed in general, (2) whether oral antibiotics are prescribed in general, and (3) whether drip antibiotics are prescribed in a visit. These three prescribing decision variables are tested against the caregivers' use of overt treatment advocacy for antibiotics variable in three tests individually. Test statistics are presented in Table 4.2.

The result reveals that a caregiver using at least one of the overt advocating actions is significantly associated with doctors' prescriptions, using the binary prescribing outcome variable of antibiotic prescriptions ($X^2 = 13.135$, $df = 1$, p < 0.001) and the binary prescribing outcome variable of drip antibiotic prescriptions ($X^2 = 21.075$, $df = 1$, p < 0.0001); however, when caregivers' use of advocating actions in the visit is tested against doctors' prescriptions of oral antibiotics, the result does not reveal significant association. These results thus indicate that although caregivers' use of overt advocating actions seems to have a significant effect on doctors' antibiotic prescription overall, such an overall effect is primarily due to the effect of caregivers' overt treatment advocacy for drip antibiotics rather than oral antibiotics.

Conclusion

In conclusion, the study's findings show that caregivers actively influence the prescribing decision by frequently advocating for antibiotic prescriptions in medical interactions. It, thus, indicates that patient/caregiver pressure is also a significant contributor to antibiotic overprescribing, similar to findings in the Western literature (Linder & Singer, 2003; Macfarlane et al., 1997; Mustafa et al., 2014; Ong et al., 2007; Scott et al., 2001). Studies from American pediatrics (Stivers, 2002a, 2005, 2007) show that caregivers can both covertly and overtly influence doctors' prescribing behavior in medical interactions. Yet, when comparing caregiver interactional behaviors in the two countries, it is found that not only do the Chinese caregivers tend to use more overt advocating actions but also use them more frequently than their American counterparts (54% vs. 9%). This finding reveals that the doctors in Chinese pediatric encounters are under a substantial amount of pressure for overprescribing, and important opportunities lie in implementing doctor training in effective response to patient caregiver pressure.

   In this chapter, I examined the interactional practices of patient caregivers to advocate for antibiotic prescriptions in medical interaction. By shifting our focus to inside the consultation room, I demonstrated how caregivers communicated their desire for antibiotics to doctors in various ways. These interactional practices put doctors under great pressure for overprescription. Statistical analyses further prove the significant impact of these interactional practices on prescription outcomes. In the next chapter, I will shift the focus to doctors' behavior in prescribing decisions. In particular, I will investigate whether doctors contribute to the problem by vigorously recommending antibiotics to their patients and whether they push caregivers to accept their recommendation by asserting a high level of authority in their interactions, as the supply-side theory suggests.

References

Britten, N. (2001). Prescribing and the defence of clinical autonomy. *Sociology of Health & Illness*, *23*(4), 478–496. https://doi.org/10.1111/1467-9566.00261

Britten, N., & Ukoumunne, O. (1997). The influence of patients' hopes of receiving a prescription on doctors' perceptions and the decision to prescribe: A questionnaire survey. *British Medical Journal*, *315*(7121), 1506–1510.

Brown, P., & Levinson, S. C. (1987). *Politeness: Some universals in language usage*. Cambridge University Press.

Choi, K.-H., Park, S.-M., Lee, J.-H., & Kwon, S. (2012). Factors affecting the prescribing patterns of antibiotics and injections. *Journal of Korean Medical Science, 27*(2), 120–127. https://doi.org/10.3346/jkms.2012.27.2.120

Curl, T. S., & Drew, P. (2008). Contingency and action: A comparison of two forms of requesting. *Research on Language and Social Interaction, 41*(2), 129–153. https://doi.org/10.1080/08351810802028613

Drew, P., & Couper-Kuhlen, E. (Eds.). (2014). *Requesting in social interaction.* John Benjamins Publishing Company.

Ervin-Tripp, S. M. (1981). How to make and understand a request. In H. Parret, M. Sbisà, & J. Verschueren (Eds.), *Possibilities and limitations of pragmatics: Proceedings of the conference on pragmatics, urbino* (p. 195). John Benjamins Publishing Company. https://doi.org/10.1075/slcs.7.13erv

Hayano, K. (2012). Question design in conversation. In *The handbook of conversation analysis* (pp. 395–414). Wiley-Blackwell. https://doi.org/10.1002/9781118325001.ch19

Heath, C. (1992). The delivery and reception of diagnosis in the general practice consultation. In *Talk at work: Interaction in institutional settings* (pp. 235–267). Cambridge University Press.

Heinemann, T. (2006). "Will you or can't you?": Displaying entitlement in interrogative requests. *Journal of Pragmatics, 38*(7), 1081–1104. https://doi.org/10.1016/j.pragma.2005.09.013

Heritage, J. (1984). A change-of-state token and aspects of its sequential placement. In *Structures of social action: Studies in conversation analysis* (pp. 299–345). Cambridge University Press.

Heritage, J. (2016). The recruitment matrix. *Research on Language and Social Interaction, 49*(1), 27–31. https://doi.org/10.1080/08351813.2016.1126440

Heritage, J., & Sefi, S. (1992). Dilemmas of advice: Aspects of the delivery and reception of advice in interactions between health visitors and first time mothers. In *Talk at Work* (pp. 3–65). Cambridge University Press.

Jefferson, G. (1981). The abominable "ne?" An exploration of post-response pursuit of response. In *Sprache der gegenwaart* (pp. 53–88). Pedagogischer Verlag Schwann.

Kendrick, K., & Drew, P. (2016). Recruitment: Offers, requests, and the organization of assistance in interaction. *Research on Language and Social Interaction, 49*(1), 1–19. https://doi.org/10.1080/08351813.2016.1126436

Kendrick, K., & Torreira, F. (2015). The timing and construction of preference: A quantitative study. *Discourse Processes, 52*(4), 255–289. https://doi.org/10.1080/0163853X.2014.955997

Li, C. N., & Thompson, S. A. (1981). *Mandarin Chinese: A functional reference grammar.* University of California Press.

Linder, J. A., & Singer, D. E. (2003). Desire for antibiotics and antibiotic prescribing for adults with upper respiratory tract infections. *Journal of General Internal Medicine, 18*(10), 795–801. https://doi.org/10.1046/j.1525-1497.2003.21101.x

Lindström, A. (2005). Language as social action: A study of how senior citizens request assistance with practical tasks in the Swedish Home Help Service. In *Syntax and Lexis in conversation* (pp. 209–230). John Benjamins.

Macfarlane, J., Holmes, W., Macfarlane, R., & Britten, N. (1997). Influence of patients' expectations on antibiotic management of acute lower respiratory tract illness in general practice: Questionnaire study. *BMJ, 315*(7117), 1211–1214. https://doi.org/10.1136/bmj.315.7117.1211

Mangione-Smith, R., Elliott, N., Stivers, T., McDonald, L., & Heritage, J. (2006). Ruling out the need for antibiotics: Are we sending the right message. *Archives of Pediatrics and Adolescent Medicine*, *160*, 945–952.

Mangione-Smith, R., McGlynn, E., Elliott, M., Krogstad, P., & Brook, R. (1999). The relationship between perceived parental expectations and pediatrician antimicrobial prescribing behavior. *Pediatrics*, *103*(4 I), 711–718.

Mangione-Smith, R., McGlynn, E., Elliott, N., McDonald, L., Franz, L., & Kravitz, L. (2001). Parent expectations for antibiotics, physician-parent communication, and satisfaction. *Archives of Pediatrics and Adolescent Medicine*, *155*(7), 800–806.

Mangione-Smith, R., Zhou, C., Robinson, J. D., Taylor, J. A., Elliott, M. N., & Heritage, J. (2015). Communication practices and antibiotic use for acute respiratory tract infections in children. *Annals of Family Medicine*, *13*(3), 221–227. https://doi.org/10.1370/afm.1785

Mustafa, M., Wood, F., Butler, C. C., & Elwyn, G. (2014). Managing expectations of antibiotics for upper respiratory tract infections: A qualitative study. *The Annals of Family Medicine*, *12*(1), 29–36. https://doi.org/10.1370/afm.1583

Ong, S., Nakase, J., Moran, G. J., Karras, D. J., Kuehnert, M. J., Talan, D. A., & EMERGEncy ID NET Study Group. (2007). Antibiotic use for emergency department patients with upper respiratory infections: Prescribing practices, patient expectations, and patient satisfaction. *Annals of Emergency Medicine*, *50*(3), 213–220. https://doi.org/10.1016/j.annemergmed.2007.03.026

Peräkylä, A. (2006). Communicating and responding to diagnosis. In *Communication in medical care: Interaction between primary care physicians and patients*. Cambridge University Press.

Pomerantz, A. (1984). *Agreeing and disagreeing with assessments: Some features of preferred/dispreferred turn shaped.* Communication Faculty Scholarship. http://scholarsarchive.library.albany.edu/cas_communication_scholar/3

Raymond, G. (2003). Grammar and social organization: Yes/no interrogatives and the structure of responding. *American Sociological Review*, *68*(6), 939–967. https://doi.org/10.2307/1519752

Reynolds, L., & Mckee, M. (2009). Factors influencing antibiotic prescribing in China: An exploratory analysis. *Health Policy*, *90*(1), 32–36.

Rossi, G. (2012). Bilateral and unilateral requests: The use of imperatives and Mi X? interrogatives in Italian. *Discourse Processes*, *49*(5), 426–458. https://doi.org/10.1080/0163853X.2012.684136

Rossi, G. (2015). *The request system in Italian.* The Max Planck Institute for Psycholinguistics & International Max Planck Research School for Language Sciences.

Scott, J. G., Cohen, D., DiCicco-Bloom, B., Orzano, A. J., Jaen, C. R., & Crabtree, B. F. (2001). Antibiotic use in acute respiratory infections and the ways patients pressure physicians for a prescription. *Journal of Family Practice*, *50*(10), 853–858.

Stivers, T. (2000). *Negotiating antibiotic treatment in pediatric care: The communication of preferences in physician-parent interaction.* University of California.

Stivers, T. (2002a). Participating in decisions about treatment: Overt parent pressure for antibiotic medication in pediatric encounters. *Social Science & Medicine*, *54*(7), 1111–1130.

Stivers, T. (2002b). "Symptoms only" and "candidate diagnoses": Presenting the problem in pediatric encounters. *Health Communication*, *3*(14), 299–338.

Stivers, T. (2005). Parent resistance to physicians' treatment recommendations: One resource for initiating a negotiation of the treatment decision. *Health Communication*, *181*(1), 41–74.

Stivers, T. (2006). The interactional process of reaching a treatment decision in acute medical encounters. In *Communication in medical care: Interactions between primary care physicians and patients* (pp. 279–312). Cambridge University Press.

Stivers, T. (2007). *Prescribing under pressure: Physician-parent conversations and antibiotics*. Oxford University Press.

Stivers, T., & Hayashi, M. (2010). Transformative answers: One way to resist a question's constraints. *Language in Society, 39*(1), 1–25. https://doi.org/10.1017/S0047404509990637

Stivers, T., Heritage, J., Barnes, R. K., McCabe, R., Thompson, L., & Toerien, M. (2017). Treatment recommendations as actions. *Health Communication*, 1–10. https://doi.org/10.1080/10410236.2017.1350913

Stivers, T., Mangione-Smith, R., Elliott, M. N., McDonald, L., & Heritage, J. (2003a). Why do physicians think parents expect antibiotics? What parents report vs what physicians believe. *The Journal of Family Practice, 52*(2), 140–147.

Stivers, T., Mangione-Smith, R., Elliott, M. N., McDonald, L., & Heritage, J. (2003b). Why do physicians think parents expect antibiotics? What parents report vs what physicians believe. *The Journal of Family Practice, 52*(2), 140–148.

Wootton, A. J. (1997). *Interaction and the development of mind*. Cambridge University Press. https://doi.org/10.1017/CBO9780511519895

5 Doctors' role in prescribing decision

Treatment recommendation actions
and medical authority in
medical visits

Introduction

In Chapter 4, my focus was on the influence of patient caregivers on prescribing decisions related to antibiotics. The findings demonstrated that in over half of the cases, the caregivers actively advocated for antibiotic prescriptions. Moreover, caregivers' advocating practices were not only observed more commonly than their American counterparts, but they were also more likely to be delivered in overt forms. These findings thus raise the question: Do doctors play no role at all in overprescription, which would be completely contradictory to the popular supply-side theory? Or do doctors now influence the problem in a more subtle manner?

In this chapter, I focus on the role of doctors in antibiotic prescribing decisions. According to the supply-side theory, if doctors were mainly driving the antibiotic overprescription problem, they would recommend antibiotic treatment for their patients whenever possible, claim a high level of authority, push for caregivers' acceptance of their antibiotic treatment recommendations, and assign caregivers a fairly passive role in the treatment decision. However, my field observation and preliminary analysis of the doctor-caregiver interaction data do not reveal this.

In the following, I will present findings related to doctors' treatment recommendations in medical encounters, specifically their content and action design. I will ask the following questions: Do doctors recommend antibiotics for their patients vigorously in medical visits? When they instigate treatment recommendation actions, do they push for caregivers' acceptance by using a high-authority and dominant conversational style? Furthermore, the preliminary analysis also shows that not all treatment plan discussions are initiated by the doctors. Instead, patient caregivers would initiate the discussion and introduce their own opinions about the treatment plan. Thus, another question to ask is: How often do caregivers initiate discussions about the treatment plan? Lastly, I will compare these findings to related findings in the American clinical context and discuss their implications for understanding the nature of the doctor–patient/caregiver relationship, which I argue is an underlying contributor to the antibiotic overprescription problem.

DOI: 10.4324/9781003243625-5

Background

Doctors' interactional practices in antibiotic prescribing interactions

A wide range of doctors' interactional practices have been found influential on antibiotic prescribing decisions in naturally occurring medical interaction.

Online commentary has been shown to be an effective way to shape parents' views of the treatment plan and reduce inappropriate antibiotic prescribing (Heritage & Stivers, 1999). This communication behavior involves the doctor describing what s/he is seeing, feeling, or hearing while examining the patient. By characterizing patient signs as mild or nonexistent (e.g., *I don't see anything in that ear* or *Her nose isn't too bad),* doctors not only indicate a 'no-problem' diagnosis and imply no need for antibiotic treatment but also reveal the grounds for this judgment (Heritage & Stivers, 1999). It is found that doctor use of this action is significantly associated with perceived parent expectations (Heritage & Stivers, 1999; Mangione-Smith et al., 2003); when doctors used 'no-problem' online commentary, they were significantly less likely to prescribe antibiotics than if they used 'problem' online commentary, citing problematic exam findings (Mangione-Smith et al., 2003). The research, thus, suggests that training doctors to more consciously and consistently apply 'no problem' online commentary in appropriate situations is most likely to reduce inappropriate antibiotic prescribing effectively, as this prepares families for a non-antibiotic treatment recommendation.

Formats of treatment recommendations also have implications for patient/ parent responses. Treatment recommendation delivery formats can be categorized into two types: (1) positive treatment recommendations – doctors' affirmative suggestions of what should be done for the patient's problem (e.g., *You can give her a teaspoonful of honey just before bedtime until the cough clears up.*) and negative recommendations – doctors' treatment recommendations against a particular treatment (e.g., *What we have here is just a virus, so antibiotics won't help.*) (Stivers, 2005a). Stivers found that doctors' use of the two treatment recommendation formats was highly consequential for parent response. She observed that negative treatment recommendations were significantly associated with parent resistance (Stivers, 2005a) and higher rates of inappropriate antibiotic prescriptions (Mangione-Smith et al., 2015), while, on the other hand, the use of positive treatment recommendations was associated with a 52% reduction in the risk of antibiotic prescribing for viral ARTIs, and the combined use of positive and negative treatment recommendations was associated with an 85% reduction in the risk of inappropriate prescribing (Mangione-Smith et al., 2015).

Additionally, *the initiator of the discussion of antibiotic treatment* is a significant indicator of patient/parent expectations for antibiotic prescriptions. It is found that parent initiation of discussions of antibiotic treatment is a significant predictor of doctors' perceptions of parental expectations for antibiotics – when parents initiate discussions about antibiotics, doctors are four times more likely to believe that they expect antibiotics than if no such initiation occurs (Mangione-Smith et al., 2001; Stivers et al., 2003). When doctors perceive parental expectations for antibiotics, they are 31.7% more likely to prescribe inappropriately (Mangione-Smith et al., 2006). Therefore, examining the distribution of the initiator of treatment discussion sheds light on the relative role of doctors and patient caregivers in the antibiotic overprescription problem.

Treatment recommendations as social actions and the doctor–patient relationship

In a study of doctors' treatment recommendations in U.S. and U.K. primary care settings, Stivers et al. (2017) systematically analyzed doctors' different treatment recommendations (i.e., pronouncements, proposals, suggestions, offers, and assertions) and found that these different actions primarily vary in the dimensions of epistemic authority and deontic authority embodied in their action design. *Epistemic authority* involves doctors' rights and power in shaping how patients view and understand a condition, primarily depending on the cultural authority of the medical profession and the achievements of scientific methods (Heritage, 2012b; Starr, 1982). *Deontic authority* involves doctors' rights and power in directing patients' future actions (Stevanovic & Peräkylä, 2012).

When delivering treatment recommendations, doctors' choice of action reflects their understanding of the extent to which they claim epistemic and deontic authority in instigating a recommendation and treatment decision-making. Pronouncements involve doctors asserting full agency over starting a recommendation, treating the decision as already determined, and as though the patient has had no choice in the matter. In contrast, offers imply doctors' willingness to prescribe medicine, treating the patient as the initiator of the recommendation and his/her preferences as an important component of the decision (Stivers et al., 2017). This denotes giving up one's sole agency over instituting the recommendation and orientation that endorsement is not required to make a decision. In sum, this analytical framework for treatment recommendation as social actions provides an important basis for us to understand the relative authority and agency that doctors and caregivers share in the doctor–patient relationship and their role in antibiotic overprescription.

Data and analytical procedures

Based on the medical conversation dataset, I examined the doctors' treatment recommendations with respect to their content and action design. Conversation analysis is used as the primary method. Each conversation was analyzed at the turn and sequence level, with a focus on how treatment recommendations are managed. Each conversation contains one or multiple treatment recommendations. Since it is common in initial recommendations for doctors and caregivers to discuss antibiotic prescriptions, I focused on the doctors' initial treatment recommendations only.

After identifying the doctors' initial treatment recommendation actions in each conversation, the actions were categorized as (1) *pronouncements*, (2) *proposals*, or (3) *offers*. The decision to consolidate the previous five classes (Stivers et al., 2018) into three was made based on the following considerations. First, because *zero anaphora* (i.e., *the* phenomenon in which pronouns fill obligatory grammatical roles such as the subject of sentences are omitted*)* is common in spoken Chinese (Chen, 1987; Li & Thompson, 1981; Tao, 1996), it is difficult to distinguish between proposals and suggestions in many cases. However, regardless of more or less weighing in on doctors' claim of agency in starting a recommendation, both actions embody a partial claim of authority and an invitation for patients' endorsement and collaboration in decision-making. I, thus, combined the two classes into one, displaying a middle level of doctors' authority in starting a treatment recommendation.

Additionally, since no instance of assertions was identified in the doctors' initial recommendations in the preliminary analysis, I removed the assertions in the three-class taxonomy. Through doing this, the consolidated three-class taxonomy is conceptualized in this way with the purpose of embodying a continuum of doctors' authority in launching a treatment recommendation and patient endorsement in the treatment recommendation actions. When classifying the treatment recommendation actions based on the three-class taxonomy, with the *pronouncements* at the highest end, the *proposals* in the middle, and the *offers* at the lowest level, the relative distribution, along with the qualitative features of the doctors' treatment recommendation actions, will provide important insights into the doctors' role in antibiotic overprescription in this setting.

Findings

Doctors' recommended treatments: antibiotics or not?

By looking at the content of the doctors' initial treatment recommendations, one can see that they do not suggest antibiotic treatment as frequently as expected. Table 5.1 outlines the distribution of the treatment that the doctors put forward in their initial recommendations.

Antibiotic treatment was proposed to patients in the doctors' initial recommendations in only 40% of the cases, whereas non-antibiotic treatment was recommended in 57% of the visits, comprising a majority. Hence, in their initial treatment recommendations, the doctors did not suggest antibiotic treatment as frequently as one would expect if they were driven primarily by financial incentives.

This observation is worth noting, particularly when compared to the proportion of antibiotic treatment that was ultimately prescribed to the patients by the end of the visit. Table 5.2 illustrates the discrepancy between the treatment initially recommended and the treatment ultimately prescribed to the patients.

As seen in the table, although antibiotics were initially recommended to the patients in 40% of the cases, they were prescribed to patients in 56% of the cases – an almost 40% increase. Given the findings that the caregivers actively participated in treatment negotiation, as shown in Chapter 4, it is likely that in at least a further 16% of the cases, the doctors' prescriptions were influenced by their interactions with caregivers.

Table 5.1 Treatment initially recommended by doctors (n=147)

Treatment*		Percentage (Frequency)	Percentage (Frequency)
Non-antibiotics			57% (n=84)
Antibiotics	Oral-antibiotics	16% (n=24)	40% (n=59)
	Drip antibiotics	24% (n=35)	
Unspecified			3% (n=4)
Total			**100% (n=147)**

Note: *Antibiotics are commonly administered through either oral medications or IV drips in this setting.
† Results are based on the cases in which the doctors initiated the initial treatment discussion (n=147).

Table 5.2 Treatment initially recommended and treatment ultimately prescribed (n=147)

Treatment	Initial recommendations		Ultimate prescriptions	
	Frequency	Percentage	Frequency	Percentage
Non-antibiotics	84	57%	65	44%
Antibiotics	59	40%	82	56%
Unspecified	4	3%		
Total	147	100%	147	100% (n=187)

Note: *In all 187 cases, patients were prescribed some specific type of treatment. In this table, I excluded 40 cases in which the treatment discussions were initiated by the patient caregivers.

Doctors' treatment recommendation actions: authoritative or not?

A second piece of evidence comes from the qualitative analysis of the doctors' treatment recommendation actions. If prescribing is supply-led, one would expect to see them pushing hard for caregivers' acceptance when they make treatment recommendations to their patients/caregivers. In the clinical setting, doctors are conventionally regarded as professionals with cultural and social authority to determine what is the best course of treatment for the patient (Freidson, 1988; Lin & Xie, 1988; Parsons, 1951; Starr, 1982); they could easily achieve this goal by asserting a high level of epistemic and deontic authority (Heritage, 2012a, 2012c; Lindström & Weatherall, 2015; Stevanovic & Peräkylä, 2012; Stevanovic & Svennevig, 2015) when delivering treatment recommendations. In other words, prescribing decisions would be presented *ex cathedra*, requiring no or little endorsement from the patients or caregivers. However, this does not seem to be the case in my dataset.

In the following, I first show a distribution of the actions that the doctors use to deliver treatment recommendations. I then go into detail to demonstrate how the doctors' choice of the action design displays their orientation toward their authority and caregivers' endorsement in treatment decision-making.

DISTRIBUTION OF THE TREATMENT RECOMMENDATION ACTIONS

As mentioned earlier, the three types of treatment recommendation actions fall on a descending scale of doctors' authority in initiating treatment recommendations and an ascending scale of patient involvement in the treatment decision. Figure 5.1 displays an illustration.

With *pronouncements*, doctors adopt a stance with both high epistemic authority and high deontic authority, leaving caregivers little room to negotiate for an alternative treatment plan (though they may still attempt this). In contrast, with *proposals* or *offers*, doctors adopt a stance where they are prepared to yield to (or at least consider) caregivers' opinions.

Thus, *pronouncements* can be considered the more authoritative treatment recommendation action, representing a higher level of agency in starting a treatment recommendation, whereas *proposals* and *offers* are presented in less authoritative terms. Table 5.3 depicts the distribution of the three types of actions that the doctors used to deliver their initial recommendations (including both antibiotic and non-antibiotic treatment) in the dataset.

As displayed in Table 5.3, doctors used the less authoritative action types (i.e., *proposals* and *offers*) more frequently than the more authoritative action type (i.e., *pronouncements*). This pattern of behavior is even more evident when doctors recommend antibiotic treatment (see Table 5.4).

Table 5.4 indicates that when doctors recommended antibiotic treatment, they used *proposals* most frequently (39% of the cases), followed by *pronouncements*

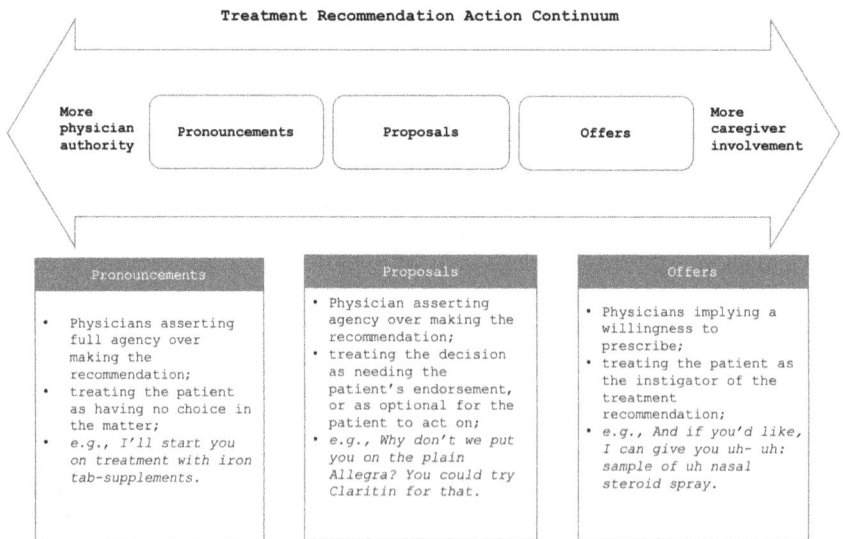

Figure 5.1 An illustration of the continuum of treatment recommendation actions

Table 5.3 Doctor-initiated treatment recommendation actions (n=147)

Actions	Frequency	Percentage
Pronouncements	61	42%
Proposals	65	44%
Offers	21	14%
Total	147	100%

Note: †Results are based on cases in which the doctors initiated the initial treatment discussion (n=147).

Table 5.4 Doctors' treatment recommendation actions and treatment recommended (n=143)*

	Non-antibiotics	Antibiotics
Pronouncements	39 (46%)	22 (37%)
Proposals	42 (50%)	23 (39%)
Offers	3 (4%)	14 (24%)
Total	**84 (100%)**†	**59 (100%)**

Note: *Among the 187 acute visits, I excluded 40 in which caregivers initiated the treatment discussion, as well as 4 in which the recommended treatment was unclear.
† Numbers in parentheses are percentages of the column totals.

(37%) and *offers* (24%). When this is compared to the U.S. primary adult care setting, we can see that doctors' antibiotic treatment recommendations in the form of *pronouncements* in the US are much more frequent, accounting for over 90% of cases (Stivers et al., 2017).

This distributional pattern suggests that (1) doctors in the Chinese pediatric setting demonstrate an overall lower level of authority than their American counterparts and (2) when doctors in the Chinese context make treatment recommendations for antibiotics, they display a lower level of authority than in their recommendations for non-antibiotic treatment. Apart from the quantitative evidence, qualitative analysis of the doctors' treatment recommendation actions provides additional support to show doctors' lower level of authority.

ACTION DESIGN OF THE TREATMENT RECOMMENDATIONS

(1) Pronouncements   are recommendations formulated in a way in which doctors assert full agency over treatment guidance, as defined in Stivers et al. (2017). The recommendation is delivered as though the decision has already been made and the caregivers have no choice in the matter. An example of a *pronouncement* in an American clinic setting is illustrated in Excerpt 5.1.

Excerpt 5.1 An example of pronouncement (US)

```
1 DOC:   O̲kay. So, (0.2) uh::m, (0.6) <I'm goi̲:ng to:>
2        start you on Ba̲ctrim,
3 DOC:   We [can do uh thre̲e day course of Bactrim,]
4 PAT:      [           ((nodding))                ]
5 DOC:   [uhm:,] =
6 PAT:   [°Okay.°/((nodding))
7 DOC:   =an:d uh: (0.2) I need tuh know how you're
8        feeling, . . .
```

This example shows a case typical of pronouncement in U.S. consultations. In this case, the doctor uses a *I'm going to do X* format to make the treatment recommendation. This turn design shows that (1) the doctor treats the treatment recommendation as a settled fact which requires no overt response or endorsement from the patient, and (2) the doctor highlights her own role in instigating the treatment recommendation. This action format thus represents a rather authoritative way that doctors deliver treatment recommendations.

In the Chinese pediatric context, this action format is also used by the doctor to deliver treatment recommendations. With the pronouncements, the doctor presents the treatment being recommended as a settled fact and caregivers' endorsement or acceptance is thus treated as not necessary. Excerpt 5.2 illustrates a case.

Excerpt 5.2 An example of pronouncement#1

Condition: Coughing
D: Doctor
GF: Grandfather

1	D:	你	是	一个	细菌性的	感染	哦.		
		ni	shi	yi-ge	xijunxingde	ganran	o		
		you	BE	one	bacterial	infection	PRT		
		"Your (condition) is a bacterial infection, OK?"							

2	GF:	哦,	细菌性	感染。					
		o,	xijunxing	ganran.					
		ok	bacterial	infection					
		"OK, a bacterial infection."							

3->	D:	细菌性	感染,	要	挂	水	的	哦.
		xijunxing	ganran	yao	gua	shui	de	o
		bacterial	infection	need	drip	fluid	ASP	PRT
		"A bacterial infection. You need to have drips."						

4	GF:	哦.
		o
		ok
		"OK."

PRT: Particle

In this case, the patient is diagnosed with a bacterial infection. After delivering the diagnosis (line 1 and line 2), the doctor makes a recommendation to put the patient on IV drip treatment (line 3). Primarily conveyed through the modal auxiliary word *yao ("*need to*")*, the recommendation is designed in a way that it states the *necessity* of using the IV drip treatment for the patient's condition rather than the possibility of choosing this treatment. More specifically, the *necessity* encompasses two dimensions: (1) it orients to the doctor's epistemic certainty regarding the treatment being recommended, based on the doctor's professional judgment of the patient's condition, and (2) it is also concerned with the social function of obligation in pushing the patient/caregiver to act in accordance with the recommendation – a deontic obligation (Bybee & Fleischman, 1995; Lyons, 1977). In sum, the action design of *pronouncement* thus displays the doctor's high level of epistemic authority and high level of deontic authority in recommending treatment.

A similar case is shown in Excerpt 5.3. In this example, the patient is visiting for persistent coughing and vomiting. In the interaction prior to the excerpt shown, the caregiver stated that before the visit, she had already given the patient some non-antibiotic medicine. After a physical examination of the patient's throat (line 1), the doctor recommends cough syrup and oral antibiotics (lines 2–3).

Excerpt 5.3 An example of pronouncement#2

Condition: Coughing, vomit
D: Doctor
M: Mother

1		((Doctor examining patient's throat))							
2->	**D:**	你	咳嗽	的话	要	加	点	咳嗽	糖浆
		ni	kesou	dehua	yao	jia	dian	kesou	tangjiang
		you	cough	case	need	add	some	cough	syrup
3		吃	吃,	加	点	消炎药	了.		
		chi	chi	jia	dian	xiaoyanyao	le		
		eat	eat	add	some	antibiotics	PRT		

"You're coughing. In that case, (you) need to add some cough syrup."

4	M:	好.
		hao
		ok

"OK."

PRT: Particle

As shown in the excerpt, the doctor's treatment recommendation also treats the decision as already made and implies that the caregiver does not have much choice in the matter. Similarly, this effect is achieved through the modal auxiliary verb *yao ("*need to*")*, which conveys the necessity of using the recommended treatment both on epistemic grounds and on deontic grounds. It, thus, also displays the doctor's high level of epistemic authority and deontic authority in the treatment decision.

Excerpt 5.4 shows another example of a doctor's *pronouncement*, in which the doctor claims an even higher level of deontic authority as compared to Excerpt 5.2. In this case, the patient is brought in for coughing and severe wheezing at the time of the visit. The doctor recommends hospital admission for the patient's condition (lines 1-2).

Excerpt 5.4 An example of pronouncement#3

Condition: Coughing, wheezing
D: Doctor
M: Mother

1->	**D:**	你	这个	必须	得	住院,	啊.
		ni	zhege	bixu	dei	zhuyuan	a
		you	this	must	ought-to	hospitalized	PRT
2		这	没啥	说	的.		
		zhe	meisha	shuo	de		
		this	nothing	say	ASP		
		"You must be hospitalized, alright? There is nothing to say."					
3	M:	住院	吧.	行.			
		zhuyuan	ba	xing			
		hospitalized	PRT	alright			
		"Hospitalized. Alright."					

ASP: Aspect marker
PRT: Particle

Similar to the doctor's treatment recommendations in Excerpt 5.2 and Excerpt 5.3, in this case, the doctor also presents the treatment recommendation as a settled matter, in which the caregiver does not have much freedom to choose. This is primarily conveyed through the lexicon choices of *bixu* ("must") and *dei* ("ought to"), two modality auxiliary verbs which not only convey the highest possible level of epistemic certainty in the speaker's judgment on the treatment plan but also the highest possible level of deontic obligation for the caregiver to act in accordance. Compared to the modal auxiliary verb *yao* ("need to") in Excerpt 5.2, although the two choices do not differ greatly in terms of the level of embodied epistemic authority, the level of embodied deontic authority is significantly higher in doctor's lexical choice of *bixu* ("must") and *dei* ("ought to") in determining the treatment. In addition, the doctor also explicitly states that "there is nothing much to say," which demarcates her stance toward the recommendation as an objective fact. This excerpt demonstrates an example of *pronouncement*, in which the doctor displays the highest level of epistemic and deontic authority in my dataset.

The previous examples show how doctor's treatment recommendations can be delivered in the format of a *pronouncement*, which treats caregivers' endorsement and participation as minimally relevant in the decision-making process. However, a detailed examination of their action design reveals that doctors commonly downgrade their epistemic and deontic authority through various mitigation devices, even in extreme cases where the doctors display their highest possible level of authority in treatment recommendations (e.g., Excerpt 5.3).

Specifically, as shown in Excerpt 5.4, although the doctor displays the highest possible level of deontic authority by using the modal auxiliary verb *bixu* *("must")*, she still appends a second TCU, *a ("alright?"),* following the treatment pronouncement (line 1), thereby reducing the forcefulness in her action design. Similarly, in Excerpt 5.3, the doctor's treatment pronouncement is also produced with mitigation devices such as (1) use of reduplicated words *chi chi ("eat eat")* and (2) prefacing the pronouncement with an evidential basis – "in the case that you are coughing"; both displaying reduced forcefulness in action design; (3) the mitigation effect can also be achieved with sentence final particles – for instance, in Excerpt 5.2, the sentence final particle *o* appended to the doctor's pronouncement also works to reduce the forcefulness of the doctor's action (Li & Thompson, 1981, p. 312).

Furthermore, omitting subject pronouns also creates an effect of mitigation. Although zero anaphora – the phenomenon that the subject pronoun of a sentence is not articulated – is common in spoken Mandarin Chinese (Chen, 1987; Li & Thompson, 1981; Tao, 1996), when subject pronouns *are* included, it displays speakers' stance toward more agency in producing their social actions. The practice has been found similarly used to achieve this effect in various languages and cultures (Ahearn, 2001; Duranti, 1988; Duranti, 2005). Therefore, compared to the doctor's *pronouncements* in Excerpt 5.3 and Excerpt 5.4, in which the subject pronoun *ni ("you")* was included in the action design, the doctor's *pronouncement* in Excerpt 5.2 displayed the doctor's mitigated assertiveness.

In sum, the doctor's *pronouncements* present the treatment recommendation as settled rather than open for discussion. This action type, thus, represents an overall authoritative format of doctor's treatment recommendation despite that they are also usually mitigated through various forms of turn design.

(2) Proposals   The second type of treatment recommendation action is the *proposal. Proposals* are recommendations produced with a reduced level of doctor's authority over treatment decisions. What primarily distinguishes *proposals* from *pronouncements* is that *proposals* explicitly invite caregivers' endorsements of the recommendation, while *pronouncements* do not. In so doing, doctors present treatment decisions as neither entirely up to them nor entirely at caregivers' discretion. Thus, the treatment decision is oriented to as a domain of shared rights and responsibilities – a collaborative endeavor between doctors and caregivers.

In the U.S. clinic settings, Stivers et al. (2017) identified two types of treatment recommendation actions that are relevant to the type of action that I describe here, including 'proposals' and 'suggestions.' According to their definitions, with 'proposals,' doctors recommend in a way that specifically invites the endorsement or collaboration of the patient, whereas with 'suggestions,' doctors recommend in a way that leaves the decision largely in the hands of the patient while, nonetheless, asserting agency over making the recommendation (Stivers et al., 2017).

Although these two actions are different in the extent to which doctors relinquish their deontic authority over the treatment decision; nevertheless, both actions are formulated as neither entirely up to the doctor nor as entirely at the patient's discretion. Moreover, since subject pronouns are often not articulated in the spoken Chinese, it is relatively difficult to separate these two actions in Mandarin (Chen, 1987; Li & Thompson, 1981; Tao, 1996). For these reasons, I combine 'proposals' and 'suggestions' into one category of treatment recommendation action, using *proposals* as a gloss for the category. Next, I provide examples of 'proposals' and 'suggestions' as defined in the U.S. clinic setting; I then illustrate doctor's *proposals* as one type of treatment recommendation action in the Chinese pediatric encounters.

Excerpt 5.5 is an example of a doctor's 'proposals' in the U.S. clinic setting. The patient presented with a severe rash and hives several days ago. The doctor recommends plain Allegra, an allergy medication, for the condition (lines 3-4).

Excerpt 5.5 An example of proposal (US)

```
 1 PAT:  . . . and that's thee only thing that was- that's
 2        d^ifferent.=[hh
 3 DOC:              [.hh Why don't we try this. (.) Why
 4        don't we put you on thuh <plain Allegra,>
 5 PAT:  Mka[y,
 7 DOC: [.hh Uh once daily dose of uh hun[dred=
 8 PAT:                                   [Kay.
 9 DOC: =an' eighty milligra:ms, an' [that should prevent=
10 PAT:                              [Mkay,
11 DOC: =this rash from coming ou:t,. . .
```

The recommendation utilizes a *proposal* format of *Why don't we*, highlighting two aspects of *proposals*: (1) it conveys the forthcoming recommendation as not yet settled but designed for further discussion, and (2) the lexical choice of *try* conveys that it is unclear whether the recommended medication will be effective in alleviating the condition, thus presenting the recommendation with an epistemic hedge and reduced deontic authority. It is argued that in contrast with *pronouncement*, where the recommendations are delivered as entirely determined at the time of delivery, the *proposal* invites collaboration in the decision-making process (Stivers et al., 2017).

Excerpt 5.6 shows a case of doctor's 'suggestions' in the U.S. clinic setting. In this case, the patient has presented with recurrent nose bleeds. Just prior to this extract, the patient has renewed complaints about nasal drainage, for which the doctor suggests Claritin, another non-antibiotic medication, as a viable treatment (line 4).

Excerpt 5.6 An example of suggestion (US)

```
1 DOC:  Theh- other possibility: i- it might be
2        just post nasal dri:p.
```

3 PAT: Well that's what ^I̲ think. you know, but:_
4 DOC: >Ya know< you could try ^Cla̲ritin for that.
5 PAT: Yeah °I've g̲o̲t some Claritin.°
6 DOC: Okay. (1.0) ((other line of questioning))

The recommendation is delivered in the format of *you could try*, highlighting two aspects of 'suggestions': (1) it highlights the patient's sole discretion in the treatment decisions, and (2) it highlights the optionality of the recommendation. Despite the fact that suggestions can take other formats, such as *I would get* or *you can try*, it is argued that all 'suggestions' treat the recommendation as optional, in direct contrast with *pronouncements* (Stivers et al., 2017).

We now turn to doctor's treatment recommendation actions in the format of *proposals* in the Chinese pediatric context. As mentioned earlier, by using *proposals*, doctors display their orientation toward the treatment decision as a collaborative endeavor and a domain of shared rights and responsibilities with the patients. In the Chinese-speaking context, this is frequently done by doctor soliciting explicit acceptance from the caregivers (e.g., using question tags such as *haoba?* ("OK?")). This contrasts with the *pronouncements*, in which the caregivers' acceptance is only normatively oriented to as relevant but not explicitly sought by the doctors as so. I illustrate this point in Excerpts 5.7–5.8.

In Excerpt 5.7, the patient has presented with coughing. The diagnostic test finds the result slightly abnormal (line 1); given this condition, the doctor recommends oral treatment for the child (line 3).

Excerpt 5.7 An example of proposal#1

Condition: Coughing
D: Doctor
GM: Grandmother

1	D:	血象	有点	高.				
		xuexiang	youdian	gao				
		hemogram	a-little	high				
		"(His) hemogram is a little high."						
2		((Four lines of discussion of child's immunity omitted))						
3->	**D:**	还好.	吃	药,	好吧?			
		haihao	chi	yao	haoba			
		alright	eat	medicine	ok			
		"It's fine. Take some oral medicine, OK?"						
4	GM:	嗯,	好.	他	喊	嘴	疼	哎.
		en	hao	ta	han	zui	teng	ai
		yeah	ok	he	shout	mouth	ache	PRT
		"Yeah, OK. He says that his mouth aches."						

PRT: Particle

As shown in the excerpt, the doctor recommends the oral treatment in a way that (1) she asserts epistemic authority over the judgment of what is the proper course of treatment for the patient's condition, yet (2) she withdraws some degree of deontic authority over the recommendation by explicitly inviting the caregiver to endorse and accept the recommended treatment (in contrast with doctors' *pronouncements*). The effect of (1) is achieved through the doctor nominating an explicit treatment plan for the patient's condition (this, in particular, is different from doctor's offers, which I will explain later). The effect of (2) is primarily conveyed through the question tag *haoba ("OK")* at the turn final, creating a conditional relevance for the caregiver's acceptance, under the sequential constraints of the question-answer adjacency pair and action type of proposal-acceptance. It, thus, displays the doctor's orientation that the treatment decision is not solely decided by him/her alone but is a joint activity in which rights and responsibilities are shared with the caregivers.

Excerpt 5.7 demonstrated a case in which the doctor displayed a relatively full epistemic authority but reduced deontic authority over his/her treatment recommendation. In the following example, I now turn to show a case in which the doctor can also retreat, at least partially, from full epistemic authority over the treatment recommendation.

In Excerpt 5.8, the patient presented with a sore throat and coughing that has lasted for two days. At line 2, the doctor recommends putting the patient on oral treatment, and the caregiver's acceptance is explicitly sought with the question tag *a* ("alright?").

Excerpt 5.8 An example of proposal#2

Condition: Sore throat, coughing
D: Doctor
M: Mother

1		((Doctor writing on medical records))							
2->	**D:**	在	家	可以	先	吃	点	药,	啊,
		zai	jia	keyi	xian	chi	dian	yao	a
		at	home	can	first	take	some	medicine	PRT
		"(You) can take some oral medicine first at home, alright?"							
3	M:	嗯.							
		en							
		yeah							
		"Yeah."							

PRT: Particle

The recommendation is formulated in a way that (1) it presents the recommendation as optional, and (2) it emphasizes the caregiver/patient's agency or discretion in the treatment decision. These two effects are primarily achieved through using the modal auxiliary verb *keyi* ("could"). The semantic meaning of *keyi* is similar to "may/might" and/or "can/could" in English. Bybee and Fleischman (1995) argue that "may/might" conveys deontic permission (*you may come in now*) and "can/could" conveys permission and root-possibility, more essentially in the domain of epistemic possibility. Following this line of reasoning, on the one hand, *keyi* ("could") highlights the 'optionality' aspect of the recommendation by presenting it as one among other options; on the other hand, it also conveys the meaning that the doctor is giving the caregiver permission to choose that treatment. Thus, the doctor's action design displays both her reduced epistemic authority and reduced deontic authority.

Moreover, the doctor downgrades her epistemic and deontic authority over the recommendation by presenting it as tentative with the lexical choice of *xian* ("first"). To further solicit the caregiver's response, the doctor also appends a question particle *a* at the turn end. Together, these turn design features show that the doctor orients to the caregivers' involvement and endorsement as essential in the treatment decision.

In sum, with recommendations in the format of a *proposal*, doctors display their recommendations as in need of caregivers' involvement and endorsement. Compared to the *pronouncements*, *proposals* display a reduction in doctors' deontic authority over the recommendation. *Pronouncements* present the recommendation as a settled decision, while *proposals* present the treatment as not yet decided. In addition, as mentioned briefly, *proposals* are also distinct from *offers* in that they maintain some epistemic authority over the recommendation, whereas *offers* do not necessarily do so. We now turn to doctors' *offers* as a third type of recommendation action in the next section.

(3) Offers　The third way for doctors to recommend treatment is to offer the treatment that caregivers desire. This action typically involves doctors inquiring about caregivers' views of their treatment preference; their views are then incorporated into the doctors' recommendations, or the caregivers may lean in to request the treatment that they desire.

Offers as an action through which treatment recommendations are delivered are also observed in the U.S. clinic setting. According to Stivers et al. (2017), what characterizes *offers* as a distinctive treatment recommendation action is that with *offers*, doctors imply a willingness to prescribe and highlight the role of patient preferences rather than medical necessity. This can be illustrated in Excerpt 5.9 – a case of an *offer* in the U.S. clinic setting.

In this case, the patient presented with ear pain. Besides an antibiotic (data not shown) and a decongestant (lines 1–2), the doctor also recommends a nasal steroid spray at lines 5–7.

Excerpt 5.9 An example of offer (US)

```
1 DOC:  And uh: for your congestion. hh I
2       would recommend taking Sudafed.
3       (.)
4 PAT:  Sudafed?=
5 DOC:  =An:d I can >if you'd li:ke< I can give you uh-
```

6   **uh: sample of uh nasal steroid spray, if you're**
7   **also really stuffy up you[r nose,**
8 PAT: [O:kay.
9 DOC: [You want that too?,=
10 PAT: [Uh huh,
11 PAT: =Ye[:s:.
12 DOC: [Okay °great.°

The recommendation is delivered in a way that highlights the occasioned nature of this recommendation by pointing to the patient's potential desire for the offered treatment with the practice *if you'd like*; addition, by using the modal auxiliary *can*, the doctor also displays the recommendation as conditional on the patient's indication of a desire for the offered treatment (Stivers et al., 2017). These features display the doctor's orientation toward the patient as the primary instigator of the recommendation. This is very similar to doctors' *offers* in the Chinese pediatric context.

Excerpts 5.10–12 illustrate three cases of doctors' *offers* in the Chinese pediatrics encounters. In Excerpt 5.10, the patient has presented with coughing. During history-taking, the caregiver stated that they had put the patient on oral medication (including non-prescribed oral antibiotics) for two days. After the caregivers evaluate the (in)effectiveness of the oral medication they had used for the child (lines 3–4), the doctor asks about whether the caregivers want to put the child on IV drip treatment (lines 5–6).

Excerpt 5.10 An example of offer#1

Condition: Coughing for two days
D: Doctor
F: Father
M: Mother

1	D:	你 ni you	这 zhe these	两 liang two	天 tian day	觉得 juede feel	吃 chi eat	的 de ASP	药 yao medicine
		"Do you feel that the medicine you took							
2		有用 youyong effective	吗? ma PRT						
		is effective?"							
3	F:	好像 haoxiang seem	效果 [xiaoguo effect	不是 bushi not	那么 name that	明显. mingxian obvious			
		"The effect seems not that obvious."							
4	M:		效果 [xiaoguo effect	不 bu not	太 tai too	明显. mingxian. obvious			

Excerpt 5.10 (Continued)

		"The effect is not too obvious."			
5->	D:	嗯. en yeah	那 na then	你 ni you	这个, zhege this	(.)
		"Yeah. Then your condition-			
6->		想 xiang want	挂 gua drip	点 dian some	水 shui fluid	啊? a PRT
		(You) want to have drip?"			
7		(1.0)				

8	F:	能 neng can	挂 gua drip	水 shui fluid	就 jiu just	挂 gua drip	点 dian some	水 shui fluid	吧. ba PRT
		"If drip is OK, then have some drip."							
	D:	嗯. en yeah *"Yeah."*							

ASP: Aspect marker
PRT: Particle

While the doctor's inquiry about the caregiver's treatment preference appears to be an understanding check of the caregivers' treatment advocacy for IV drip treatment conveyed through their negative evaluations of the oral treatment, it also indicates the doctor's willingness to prescribe. In response, the caregiver provides a transformative answer (Stivers & Hayashi, 2010), switching the agenda of the doctor's turn by directly requesting the offered treatment. As shown in this case, the doctor's *offer* thus displays a relinquishment of her epistemic and deontic authority over the treatment decision, as the recommendation is primarily made to cater to the caregivers' desires.

Excerpt 5.11 illustrates a similar case. In this excerpt, the patient has presented with recurrent coughing during the past month. The doctor suggests the patient take an X-ray test to see if there is pneumonia (line 2); the caregiver rejects the diagnostic test recommendation (lines 3–11). Subsequently, the doctor offers a treatment recommendation by asking about the caregiver's treatment preferences (line 13).

Excerpt 5.11 An example of offer#2

Condition: coughing
D: Doctor
M: Mother

1		((A few lines of X-ray test recommendation omitted))					
2	D:	你 ni	还 hai	想 xiang	拍 pai	个 ge	片子 pianzi	啊? a

(Continued)

Excerpt 5.11 (Continued)

		you	still	want	take	CT	photo	PRT

"You still want to take an (X-ray) photo?"

3   (1.0)

4   M:
拍	片子	啊?
pai	pianzi	a
take	photo	PRT

"Take a photo?"

5   (1.8)

6   M:
拍	片子	是	什么?	那个	X光	的,
pai	pianzi	shi	shenme	nage	X-guang	de
take	photo	is	what	that	X-Ray	ASP

"Take a photo, what is it? That X-ray photo?"

7   D:
对.
dui
right
'Right.'

8   M:
要不	算了	先.
yaobu	suanle	xian
or	forget-it	first

"Or (we) won't do it first."

9   D:
暂时	先	[不	拍.
zanshi	xian	bu	pai
temporary	first	not	take

"(You) don't take it for the moment?"

10   M:
[嗯,	先	不	拍.
en	xian	bu	pai
yeah	first	not	take

"Yeah, we won't take it first."

11   D:
行。
xing
alright
"Alright."

12   (2.6)

13->   **D:**
你	想	怎么样	啊?
ni	xiang	zenmeyang	a
you	want	what	PRT

"What do you want?

14
想	挂	水	还是	吃	药	啊?
xiang	gua	shui	haishi	chi	yao	a
want	drip	fluid	or	eat	medicine	PRT

(Do you) want to have drips or take oral medicine?"

15   M:
嗯:,	你	看	这个,	现在	吃	的话,
en	ni	kan	zhege	xianzai	chi	dehua
yeah	you	look	zthis	now	eat	case

"Yeah, in your opinion, if (we) take oral medicine now,

16
[这个	药-
zhege	yao
this	medicine

this medicine-"

(Continued)

Excerpt 5.11 (Continued)

17	D:	[现在	没有	用	了.
		xianzai	meiyou	yong	le
		now	no	use	ASP
		"It's no use now."			

CT: Count
PRT: Particle
ASP: Aspect marker

The doctor's *offer* is formulated in a way that casts the caregiver's role as central to the treatment decision. This is done first by asking an open-ended question about what the caregiver wants for treatment – *what do you want?* – and second, by using an alternative question to invite the caregiver to choose from the two options presented – *(do you) want to have drips or oral medication?*

It should be noted that compared to the doctor's *offer* in Excerpt 5.10, the doctor's *offer* in the open-ended question and the alternative question format embodies a further downgrading of the doctor's epistemic and deontic authority. With the polar question, the doctor nominates one treatment and thus at least weakly endorses it by allowing the caregiver to confirm and decide, whereas the doctor's alternative question and open-ended question displays no endorsement for any particular treatment at all. Consequently, the caregiver is given the full responsibility to the treatment decision.

Excerpt 5.12 presents another case of a doctor's *offer*, in which the doctor uses only an open-ended question to ask about the caregiver's treatment preference. In this case, the patient has presented with a fever and cough over the past few days. In lines 1 to 5, the doctor takes the patient's medication history and the caregiver states that she has given the patient non-prescribed oral antibiotics for two to three days prior to the visit. Subsequently, the doctor produces an understanding check as to whether the oral antibiotics have not been effective (line 7) and what the mother wants to have for the patient's condition (line 8). Subsequently, the mother states her preference for an IV antibiotic treatment despite that it is mitigated in an inquiry delivery format – *Does this need drip?* Learning about the mother's opinion, the doctor then recommends putting the patient on an antibiotic IV treatment.

Excerpt 5.12 An example of offer#3

Condition: Fever, cough for two days
M: Mother
D: Doctor

1	M:	消炎	药	我	在	家	也
		xiaoyan	yao	wo	zai	jia	ye
		antibiotic	medicine	I	at	home	also

Excerpt 5.12 (Continued)

		"Oral antibiotics, I also gave him					
2		给	他	吃	的.		
		gei	ta	chi	de		
		give	him	eat	ASP		
		some to take at home."					
3	D:	吃	的	什么	啊?		
		chi	de	shenme	a		
		eat	PRT	what	PRT		
		"What did you give him to take?"					
4	M:	头孢.					
		toubao					
		cephalo					
		"Cephalo."					
5	D:	吃	了	几	天	啊?	
		chi	le	ji	tian	a	
		eat	ASP	many	day	PRT	
		"How many days has he taken?"					
6	M:	吃	了	两	三	天.	
		chi	le	liang	san	tian	
		eat	ASP	two	three	day	
		"(He's) taken it for two or three days."					
7=>	**D:**	不	管用	是	啊?		
		bu	guanyong	shi	a		
		not	work	BE	PRT		
		"Not working, is it?					
8=>		那	你	想	怎么	呢?	
		na	ni	xiang	zenme	ne	
		then	you	want	what	PRT	
		Then what do you want?"					
9->	**M:**	这	要	挂	水	吧?	
		zhe	yao	gua	shui	ba	
		this	need	drip	fluid	PRT	
		"Does this need drip?"					
10=>	**D:**	挂	点	吧,	好	吧?	
		gua	dian	ba	hao	ba	
		drip	some	PRT	ok	PRT	
		"Have some drip, OK?					
11=>		别	往	气管	发展	了.	
		bie	wang	qiguan	fazhan	le	
		don't	toward	trachea	develop	ASP	
		Don't let it develop toward the trachea."					
12	M:	那	就	给	他	挂	下	吧.
		na	jiu	gei	ta	gua	xia	ba
		then	just	give	him	drip	time	PRT
		"Then let's just put him on drip, OK?					
13		看	他	这	两	天	咳	得
		kan	ta	zhe	liang	tian	ke	de
		see	him	these	two	day	cough	ASP
		I see him coughing					

(Continued)

Excerpt 5.12 (Continued)

14	太	厉害	了.
	tai	lihai	le
	too	bad	ASP
	too bad these two days."		

ASP: Aspect marker
PRT: Particle

With the open-ended question format *What do you want?*, the doctor avoids presenting any option to the caregiver. Compared to the alternative question in Excerpt 5.11 and the polar question in Excerpt 5.10, the open-ended format of the *offer* is less restrictive, thus allowing the caregiver to state her preference openly. Despite these subtle differences, the doctor's *offers* indicate a willingness to accommodate the caregiver's preferences. Therefore, the treatment decision is oriented to be not solely based on medical appropriateness but also, and perhaps more importantly, on the patient or caregiver's personal preferences.

Moreover, besides deploying the syntactic structure of a question in exploring caregivers' treatment preferences, what is also common to the doctors' *offers* is that in these cases, the doctors uniformly appeal to the caregivers' *wants* or *desires* in the recommendation actions. In the three excerpts shown, the lexicon choice of *xiang* ("want/desire") are all present. This turn design feature thus characterizes the doctors' *offers* as primarily based on caregivers' indications of preferences and desires for treatment rather than medical necessity and appropriateness.

These examples, thus, show that with *offers*, doctors orient to caregivers' sole responsibilities in treatment decision-making. Compared to *proposals*, in which doctors orient to their responsibilities as shared with caregivers, *offers* display doctors' downgraded epistemic authority and abdication of deontic authority in treatment decisions. Compared to *pronouncements*, in which doctors take the primary responsibility in treatment decision-making and present the treatment decision as settled, *offers* stand in direct contrast. Therefore, doctors' *offers* display their lowest epistemic and deontic authority over the treatment decision, and the decision is primarily based on caregivers' preferences.

Taken together, these examples show that with *offers*, doctors orient themselves toward caregivers' primary responsibility in treatment decision-making. Compared to *proposals*, in which doctors focus on their responsibilities as shared with caregivers, *offers* display the doctors' downgraded epistemic authority and relinquishment of deontic authority in treatment decisions. Compared to *pronouncements*, in which doctors take primary responsibility in treatment decision-making and present the treatment as settled with minimal patient involvement, *offers* stand in direct contrast. Therefore, doctors' choice of action design indicates their lowest epistemic and deontic authority over the treatment decision.

Although only accounting for a relatively small portion, the doctors' *offer* of treatment recommendations displays their orientation to caregiver preferences as important in treatment decisions, even for prescription medicine such as antibiotics, for which doctors should act as gatekeepers and be stringent in prescribing. The fact that doctors tend to deploy low-authority communication styles such as *offers* and *proposals* indicates that they may be concerned more about the satisfaction of the caregivers than the appropriateness of the prescription. In cases where cautious prescribing is required, they may not be willing to make a compromise on patient/caregiver satisfaction (O'Connor et al., 2018).

The tendency to provide patients/caregivers with what they desire reflects the doctor–patient relationship that underlies the observed behavioral pattern. In this type of relationship, doctors do not assert their high level of medical authority, while patients assert a high level of agency and entitlement in treatment decision-making. When compared to doctors' prescribing style in the American clinic context, doctors in the Chinese context demonstrated an overall lower level of medical authority in treatment decision-making. The rather egalitarian relationship between doctors and caregivers, thus, indicates that when making treatment recommendations in this clinic setting, the Chinese doctors are not relying on their medical authority to facilitate caregivers' acceptance of any particular treatment, including the antibiotic treatment. However, such an egalitarian relationship might also give way to the caregivers' higher-frequency and more overt forms of treatment advocacy for antibiotics, which is indirectly linked to the overprescription in this clinic setting.

Besides the action design of the doctor's treatment recommendation, examining how frequently caregivers initiate treatment discussions also sheds light on this doctor–patient relationship and its impact on antibiotic overprescription.

Who initiates the treatment discussion – Doctors or caregivers?

The patient caregiver's initiation of a discussion about antibiotic treatment significantly affects doctors' perception of parental expectations for antibiotics. This, in turn, increases the likelihood of inappropriate prescriptions. In a sample of American pediatric encounters, when parents initiated discussions about antibiotics, doctors were four times more likely to believe that they expected antibiotics than if no such initiation had occurred (Mangione-Smith et al., 2001). When doctors perceived parental expectations for antibiotics, they were 31.7% more likely to prescribe inappropriately (Mangione-Smith et al., 2006). Examining the frequency and method by which patient caregivers initiate treatment discussions also sheds important light on the relative role of doctors and caregivers in antibiotic prescriptions.

The data show that although treatment recommendations are conventionally considered within the domain of doctors' professional expertise, Chinese caregivers take a highly agentive role in discussing treatment plans and influencing treatment decisions. Table 5.5 illustrates the distribution of the initiator of the treatment discussion and the recommended treatment.

This finding shows that caregivers took the initiative to discuss treatment plans in 21% of the visits in the dataset. This percentage is high, given that treatment plans are conventionally oriented toward the domain of doctors' expertise.

Table 5.5 Initiator of the treatment discussion and the treatment recommended (n=187)

Initiator	Treatment	Frequency	(%)	Percentage
Doctor		147		79%
Caregiver	Antibiotics	21	(53%)	
	Non-antibiotics	18	(45%)	
	Unspecified	1	(2%)	
	Subtotal	40	(100%)	21%
Total		187		100%

Moreover, in over half of the cases, the patient-initiated treatment discussion involved antibiotics.

This contrasts with the findings in the American pediatric encounters – doctors initiated discussions of antibiotic treatment 74% of the time, whereas parents initiated these conversations 8% of the time (Mangione-Smith et al., 2001). As mentioned previously, when patient caregivers started the discussion of antibiotic treatment, doctors were more likely to perceive them as expecting antibiotic prescriptions and were thus more likely to prescribe inappropriately. I illustrate this point in the following section.

DESIGN AND DELIVERY OF CAREGIVER-INITIATED TREATMENT
RECOMMENDATIONS

In the previous subsections, I showed that when doctors initiate treatment recommendations, they tend to use less authoritative forms of actions, and the majority of their treatment recommendations are for non-antibiotics (57%–60%). Despite varying in their degree of endorsement and authority embodied in their action designs, these recommendations are all initiated by doctors; nevertheless, in 21% of the visits in my dataset, caregivers initiate the discussion of treatment plans. In this section, I focus on the treatment discussions that are initiated by the caregivers. My point is that although treatment recommendations are conventionally considered to be within the domain of doctors' professional expertise, caregivers, in many cases, take the initiative to discuss treatment options and thus display their orientation as having the right to influence doctors' prescribing behaviors. In the following, I first illustrate two examples of such caregiver-initiated treatment discussions; I then show how frequently these discussions are about antibiotics.

Excerpt 5.13 illustrates a case of a caregiver-initiated discussion of treatment plans. In this case, the patient presented with a cough and fever over the past two days. After a physical examination, the doctor takes the history of the patient's symptoms in more detail (not shown in the data). After some extensive detailing of the patient's symptoms by the two caregivers (lines 2–3), the caregiver initiates the discussion of the treatment plan by inquiring about IV drip treatment (line 5). The inquiry is understood by the doctor as overtly advocating for the IV treatment; following the inquiry, the doctor offers to prescribe the IV treatment (line 8).

Excerpt 5.13 An example of a caregiver-initiated treatment discussion#1

Condition: Coughing, fever for two days
M: Mother
GM: Grandmother

1		((A few lines of discussion of the patient's cough omitted))				
2	**M:**	都	蛮	凶的,	半夜	都	咳.
		dou	man	xiongde	banye	dou	ke
		all	rather	bad	mid-night	all	cough

"(He) coughed rather bad both day and night.
He coughed even in the middle of the night."

3	GM:	都	咳,	反正	都	咳.
		dou	ke	fanzheng	dou	ke
		all	cough	anyway	all	cough

"He coughed day and night. He coughed all the time anyway."

4		(2.2)				
5=>	**M:**	他	要	挂	水	吧?
		Ta	yao	gua	shui	ba
		He	need	drip	fluid	PRT

"Does he need drip?"

6->	**D:**	今天	要么	就	给	你	挂	水	啊?
		jintian	yaome	jiu	gei	ni	gua	shui	a
		today	otherwise	just	give	you	drip	fluid	PRT

"Otherwise let me give you some drip today, OK?"

PRT: Particle

The doctor's offer of the IV treatment is delivered in a way that it clearly registers it as occasioned by the caregivers' treatment advocacy. This is primarily conveyed through the lexicon choice *yaome* ("otherwise"), which has the meaning of conditionality, or even concession, dependent on the caregiver's action. Thus, as shown in the example, when caregivers initiate the discussion of treatment plans, they put doctors in a position to address whatever stance they take toward the treatment.

Excerpt 5.14 illustrates another example in which the caregiver initiates the treatment recommendation ahead of the doctor. In this case, the patient has presented with a cold over the past week and fever during the last night. Through lines 1 to 3, the doctor first delivers a viral cold diagnosis of the child's condition (line 1); this is followed by the mother's resistance (Stivers, 2005b) at line 2. In the face of the caregiver's diagnosis resistance, the doctor further supports it by explicating the details of the test results and by concluding that it is – *Nothing serious.* (lines 3–6). Following this, the caregiver initiates the discussion of the treatment plan, asking whether an antibiotic IV treatment is needed (line 7).

Excerpt 5.14 An example of patient-initiated treatment discussion#2

Condition: Cold for a week, fever last night
D: Doctor
M: Mother

1	D:	还	是	病毒	感冒.	
		hai	shi	bingdu	ganmao	
		still	BE	viral	cold	
		"(It's) still a viral cold."				
2	M:	病毒	感冒,	是	啊?	
		bingdu	ganmao	shi	a	
		biral	cold	BE	PRT	
		"A viral cold, is it?"				
3	D:	对	对	对.		
		dui	dui	dui		
		right	right	right		
		"Right, right right.				
4		白细胞	种类	中性	都	正常,
		baixibao	zhonglei	zhongxing	dou	zhengchang
		white cell	type	neutral	all	normal
		White cell type and neutral are all normal.				
5		就是	C反应	蛋白	稍微	高	一点点.
		jiushi	C-fanying	danbai	shaowei	gao	yidiandian
		just	C-reactive	protein	slightly	high	a little
		Just the C-reactive protein is slightly high.					
6		没	啥	说法.		
		mei	sha	shuofa		
		no	what	saying		
		Nothing serious."				
7=>	**M:**	要	挂	水	吗?	
		yao	gua	shui	ma	
		need	drip	fluid	PRT	
		"(Does he) need drip?"				
8	D:	可以	不	挂.	吃	药.
		keyi	bu	gua	chi	yao
		can	not	drip	eat	medicine
		"Drip can be optional. Take some oral medicine."				
9	M:	哦,	行.			
		o	xing			
		ok	alright			
		"OK, alright."				

PRT: Particle

In response to the caregiver's question, the doctor first answers – *You could have no drip*; this is then followed with a positive-format recommendation to put the patient on oral treatment (line 8). It should be noted that the doctor displays herself as under pressure following the caregiver's initiation of the treatment discussion. This can be evidenced by the doctor's choice of modal auxiliary verb *keyi* ("could"). By using this word, the doctor presents the negative-format recommendation as optional for the patient. Although the negative-format treatment recommendation is immediately appended with a positive-format recommendation for the oral treatment, the optionality conveyed through the doctor's turn design still opens the possibility for the caregiver to negotiate for the antibiotic IV treatment.

Excerpt 5.15 illustrates a similar case of caregiver-initiated discussion of treatment plans. The patient is brought in for coughing during the night. After a physical examination of the patient's throat, the doctor delivers a tentative diagnosis of the patient's condition at line 1. Following this tentative diagnosis, the caregiver initiates the discussion of the treatment plan at line 3.

Excerpt 5.15 An example of patient-initiated treatment discussion#3

Condition: Coughing for one night
D: Doctor
M: Mother

1	D:	可能	还	是	支气管	有	问题.
		keneng	hai	shi	zhiqiguan	you	wenti
		perhaps	still	BE	bronchia	have	problem
		"Perhaps it's still something wrong with the bronchia."					

2		(1.0)					
3->	**M:**	挂	点	水.			
		gua	dian	shui			
		drip	some	fluid			
		"Have some drip."					

4	D:	不	要	挂	水	吧,	
		bu	yao	gua	shui	ba	
		no	need	drip	fluid	PRT	
		"No need for drip, OK?					

5		你	又不	发烧,	好	吧?	
		ni	youbu	fashao	hao	ba	
		you	not	fever	ok	PRT	
		You don't have any fever, OK?"					

6	M:	不	挂	水	不	行	啊,
		bu	gua	shui	bu	xing	a
		not	drip	fluid	not	alright	PRT
		"It won't work if he doesn't have drip.					

7		吃	药	吃	了		
		chi	yao	chi	le		
		eat	medicine	eat	ASP		
		He's taken oral medicine					

8		两	天	不	行	哎.	
		liang	tian	bu	xing	ai	
		two	day	not	alright	PRT	
		for two days, and it didn't work."					

Excerpt 5.15 (Continued)

9	D:	我	建议	你	还是	吃-	吃	点	阿奇霉素.
		wo	jianyi	ni	haishi	chi	chi	dian	aqimeisu
		I	suggest	you	still	eat	eat	some	azithromycin.
		"I suggest you still take some oral azithromycin."							

PRT: Particle

The caregiver's initiation of the treatment discussion is formulated in the form of a request for an antibiotic IV treatment. Since the explicit request is the most overt and imposing type of caregiver advocating action, it puts the doctor under pressure to prescribe the treatment. Nevertheless, even in the face of such an overt from of treatment advocacy (lines 4–5), the doctor here rejects the caregiver's request. It should be noted that although the doctor rejects the request, she still displays herself as under pressure. First, in response to the request, the doctor formulates her turn with a transformative answer, changing the original agenda of the caregiver's turn from granting/rejecting the request to assessing the need for the requested treatment (lines 4). Second, the transformative answer is also produced with a final particle *ba*, working to reduce the forcefulness of the action. Third, the doctor accounts for her rejection by providing a rationale as to why the requested treatment is not needed (line 5) – *You don't have fever.*

In this case, following the doctor's rejection of the request, the caregiver again advocates for the IV drip treatment by using a second overt advocating strategy – delivering a negative evaluation of the oral treatment (lines 6–8). Despite the caregiver's continued pressure for the IV drip prescription, the doctor maintains her original stance, by changing to offer a positive-format recommendation for oral treatment (line 9). Nonetheless, it is noted that her re-offering of the oral treatment nominates azithromycin, an oral antibiotic, as the primary medicine; in addition, the lexicon choice of *haishi* ("still") demarcates her stance as in conflict with the caregiver's. This choice shows that the doctor's offering of the oral antibiotic is at least partially due to the caregiver's pressure for prescribing.

In sum, across the dataset, the caregivers initiated the treatment discussion in 21% of the cases (n=40); among them, more than half were caregivers bidding for antibiotic treatment. These results, therefore, suggest further that in a context where the doctors and caregivers are oriented toward a rather even distribution of rights and responsibilities in treatment decision-making, the caregivers demonstrate a high level of agency and entitlement in obtaining antibiotic prescriptions, even though treatment plans are conventionally regarded as being within the domain of the doctors' professional expertise. Although doctors generally do not vigorously recommend antibiotics, their relinquishment of professional authority in prescribing decisions and the nature of their relationship with caregivers at least partially contribute to the high prevalence of antibiotic overprescription.

Conclusion

The findings of this chapter suggest that contrary to the supply-side theory that doctors are driving the antibiotic overprescription problem because of perverse incentives, the role of doctors in the problem is changing. Evidence from the naturally occurring doctor-caregiver conversation data shows that (1) the doctors did not recommend antibiotics as much as expected, (2) the doctors did not promote antibiotics by mandating caregivers' acceptance and displaying a high level of authority in their treatment recommendation action, and (3) even though it is not within their domain of expertise, the caregivers initiated discussion of treatment plans in a considerably large proportion of the visits, of which a majority involved antibiotics. Therefore, the high prevalence of antibiotic prescription is not down to doctors vigorously marketing to their patients but, instead, is a consequence of the current mode of relationship between doctors and patients/caregivers and the patterns of interaction that come with it.

These findings highlight the social dimensions of prescribing practices in clinical settings (Dixon et al., 2021; Kronman et al., 2020; Mangione-Smith et al., 2015; Stivers, 2007; Willis & Chandler, 2019). First, rather than being solely determined based on doctors' judgment of its medical appropriateness, prescribing decisions and the recommendation of the treatment are influenced by doctors' perception of the caregivers' expectations and preferences. Second, rather than being treated as a static outcome, prescribing decisions should be understood as an interactional achievement. Doctors' treatment recommendations are delivered in a way that takes into account the willingness of the caregivers and the likelihood of their acceptance.

Lastly, the way prescribing decisions are made and how treatment recommendations are delivered are also influenced by the level of authority that doctors assert in the doctor–patient relationship. As shown in this chapter, when compared to doctors' treatment recommendation actions in contemporary American, British, and Japanese clinical practices (Barnes, 2018; Bergen et al., 2018; Kushida & Yamakawa, 2015; Landmark et al., 2015, Stivers, 2007; Stivers & Timmermans, 2020; Toerien et al., 2011), the level of professional authority of Chinese doctors is considerably lower. When doctors do not assume a high level of professional authority, they display a tendency to accommodate the patients' desires and preferences in prescribing decisions. Relatedly, when the patients do not defer to the doctors' professional authority, they display a high level of entitlement and agency in medical decisions, even though their desires and preferences may not always be medically appropriate.

In a survey study, He (2014) argued that the excessive use of diagnostic tests and prescriptions in China was partly due to doctors engaging in defensive medicine to avoid disputes with their patients in the context of a tensioned doctor–patient relationship (Tucker et al., 2016; Wang et al., 2012). The study's finding corroborates this theory. In the next chapter, I will examine the relative roles of doctors and patient caregivers in the problem of antibiotic overprescription. I will investigate their interactive behavior in the conversational sequence (Schegloff, 2007) of treatment recommendation-response.

References

Ahearn, L. M. (2001). Language and agency. *Annual Review of Anthropology*, *30*, 109–137.
Barnes, R. K. (2018). Preliminaries to treatment recommendations in UK primary care: A vehicle for shared decision making? *Health Communication*, *33*(11), 1366–1376. https://doi.org/10.1080/10410236.2017.1350915

Bergen, C., Stivers, T., Barnes, R. K., Heritage, J., McCabe, R., Thompson, L., & Toerien, M. (2018). Closing the deal: A cross-cultural comparison of treatment resistance. *Health Communication*, *33*(11), 1377–1388. https://doi.org/10.1080/10410236.2017.1350917

Bybee, J. L., & Fleischman, S. (1995). *Modality in grammar and discourse*. John Benjamins Publishing Company. https://benjamins.com/catalog/tsl.32

Chen, P. (1987). Hanyu Lingxing Huizhi de Huayu Fenxi. *Zhongguo Yuwen*, *5*(200).

Dixon, J., Manyau, S., Kandiye, F., Kranzer, K., & Chandler, C. I. R. (2021). Antibiotics, rational drug use and the architecture of global health in Zimbabwe. *Social Science & Medicine*, *272*, 113594. https://doi.org/10.1016/j.socscimed.2020.113594

Duranti, A. (1988). Intentions, language, and social action in a Samoan context. *Journal of Pragmatics*, *12*(1), 13–33. https://doi.org/10.1016/0378-2166(88)90017-3

Duranti, A. (2005). Agency in language. In A. Duranti (Ed.), *A companion to linguistic anthropology* (pp. 449–473). Blackwell Publishing Ltd. https://doi.org/10.1002/9780470996522.ch20

Freidson, E. (1988). *Profession of medicine: A study of the sociology of applied knowledge*. University of Chicago Press.

He, A. J. (2014). The doctor–patient relationship, defensive medicine and overprescription in Chinese public hospitals: Evidence from a cross-sectional survey in Shenzhen city. *Social Science & Medicine*, *123*, 64–71. https://doi.org/10.1016/j.socscimed.2014.10.055

Heritage, J. (2012a). Epistemics in action: Action formation and territories of knowledge. *Research on Language and Social Interaction*, *45*(1), 1–29. https://doi.org/10.1080/0835 1813.2012.646684

Heritage, J. (2012b). Epistemics in conversation. In *The handbook of conversation analysis* (pp. 370–394). Wiley-Blackwell. https://doi.org/10.1002/9781118325001.ch18

Heritage, J. (2012c). The epistemic engine: Sequence organization and territories of knowledge. *Research on Language and Social Interaction*, *45*(1), 30–52. https://doi.org/10.108 0/08351813.2012.646685

Heritage, J., & Stivers, T. (1999). Online commentary in acute medical visits: A method of shaping patient expectations. *Social Science & Medicine (1982)*, *49*(11), 1501–1517.

Kronman, M. P., Gerber, J. S., Grundmeier, R. W., Zhou, C., Robinson, J. D., Heritage, J., Stout, J., Burges, D., Hedrick, B., Warren, L., Shalowitz, M., Shone, L. P., Steffes, J., Wright, M., Fiks, A. G., & Mangione-Smith, R. (2020). Reducing antibiotic prescribing in primary care for respiratory illness. *Pediatrics*, *146*(3). https://doi.org/10.1542/peds.2020-0038

Kushida, S., & Yamakawa, Y. (2015). Fitting proposals to their sequential environment: A comparison of turn designs for proposing treatment in ongoing outpatient psychiatric consultations in Japan. *Sociology of Health & Illness*, *37*(4), 522–544. https://doi.org/10.1111/1467-9566.12204

Landmark, A. M. D., Gulbrandsen, P., & Svennevig, J. (2015). Whose decision? Negotiating epistemic and deontic rights in medical treatment decisions. *Journal of Pragmatics*, *78*, 54–69. https://doi.org/10.1016/j.pragma.2014.11.007

Li, C. N., & Thompson, S. A. (1981). *Mandarin Chinese: A functional reference grammar*. University of California Press.

Lin, N., & Xie, W. (1988). Occupational prestige in urban China. *American Journal of Sociology*, *93*(4), 793–832. JSTOR.

Lindström, A., & Weatherall, A. (2015). Orientations to epistemics and deontics in treatment discussions. *Journal of Pragmatics*, *78*(suppl_C), 39–53. https://doi.org/10.1016/j.pragma.2015.01.005

Lyons, J. (Ed.). (1977). Deixis, space and time. In *Semantics* (Vol. 2, pp. 636–724). Cambridge University Press. https://doi.org/10.1017/CBO9780511620614.008

Mangione-Smith, R., Elliott, N., Stivers, T., McDonald, L., & Heritage, J. (2006). Ruling out the need for antibiotics: Are we sending the right message. *Archives of Pediatrics and Adolescent Medicine, 160*, 945–952.

Mangione-Smith, R., McGlynn, E., Elliott, N., McDonald, L., Franz, L., & Kravitz, L. (2001). Parent expectations for antibiotics, physician-parent communication, and satisfaction. *Archives of Pediatrics and Adolescent Medicine, 155*(7), 800–806.

Mangione-Smith, R., Stivers, T., Elliott, N., McDonald, L., & Heritage, J. (2003). Online commentary during the physical examination: A communication tool for avoiding inappropriate antibiotic prescribing? *Social Science & Medicine, 56*(2), 313–320.

Mangione-Smith, R., Zhou, C., Robinson, J. D., Taylor, J. A., Elliott, M. N., & Heritage, J. (2015). Communication practices and antibiotic use for acute respiratory tract infections in children. *Annals of Family Medicine, 13*(3), 221–227. https://doi.org/10.1370/afm.1785

O'Connor, R., O'Doherty, J., O'Regan, A., & Dunne, C. (2018). Antibiotic use for acute respiratory tract infections (ARTI) in primary care; what factors affect prescribing and why is it important? A narrative review. *Irish Journal of Medical Science (1971 -), 187*(4), 969–986. https://doi.org/10.1007/s11845-018-1774-5

Parsons, T. (1951). *Social system.* Routledge.

Schegloff, E. (2007). *Sequence organization in interaction: A primer in conversation analysis.* Cambridge University Press.

Starr, P. (1982). *The social transformation of American medicine: The rise of a Sovereign profession and the making of a vast industry.* Basic Books.

Stevanovic, M., & Peräkylä, A. (2012). Deontic authority in interaction: The right to announce, propose, and decide. *Research on Language & Social Interaction, 45*(3), 297–321. https://doi.org/10.1080/08351813.2012.699260

Stevanovic, M., & Svennevig, J. (2015). Introduction: Epistemics and deontics in conversational directives. *Journal of Pragmatics, 78*, 1–6. https://doi.org/10.1016/j.pragma.2015.01.008

Stivers, T. (2005a). Non-antibiotic treatment recommendations: Delivery formats and implications for parent resistance. *Social Science & Medicine, 5*(60), 949–964.

Stivers, T. (2005b). Parent resistance to physicians' treatment recommendations: One resource for initiating a negotiation of the treatment decision. *Health Communication, 181*(1), 41–74.

Stivers, T. (2007). *Prescribing under pressure: Physician-parent conversations and antibiotics.* Oxford University Press.

Stivers, T., & Hayashi, M. (2010). Transformative answers: One way to resist a question's constraints. *Language in Society, 39*(1), 1–25. https://doi.org/10.1017/S0047404509990637

Stivers, T., Heritage, J., Barnes, R. K., McCabe, R., Thompson, L., & Toerien, M. (2017). Treatment recommendations as actions. *Health Communication*, 1–10. https://doi.org/10.1080/10410236.2017.1350913

Stivers, T., Heritage, J., Barnes, R. K., McCabe, R., Thompson, L., & Toerien, M. (2018). Treatment recommendations as actions. *Health Communication, 33*(11), 1335–1344. https://doi.org/10.1080/10410236.2017.1350913

Stivers, T., Mangione-Smith, R., Elliott, M. N., McDonald, L., & Heritage, J. (2003). Why do physicians think parents expect antibiotics? What parents report vs what physicians believe. *The Journal of Family Practice, 52*(2), 140–148.

Stivers, T., & Timmermans, S. (2020). Medical authority under siege: How clinicians transform patient resistance into acceptance. *Journal of Health and Social Behavior, 61*(1), 60–78. https://doi.org/10.1177/0022146520902740

Tao, H. (1996). *Units in Mandarin conversation.* John Benjamins Publishing Company. https://benjamins.com/#catalog/books/sidag.5/main

Doctors' role in prescribing decision 89

Toerien, M., Shaw, R., Duncan, R., & Reuber, M. (2011). Offering patients choices: A pilot study of interactions in the seizure clinic. *Epilepsy & Behavior*, *20*(2), 312–320. https://doi.org/10.1016/j.yebeh.2010.11.004

Tucker, J. D., Wong, B., Nie, J.-B., & Kleinman, A. (2016). Rebuilding patient–physician trust in China. *The Lancet*, *388*(10046), 755. https://doi.org/10.1016/S0140-6736(16)31362-9

Wang, X.-Q., Wang, X.-T., & Zheng, J.-J. (2012). How to end violence against doctors in China. *The Lancet*, *380*(9842), 647–648. https://doi.org/10.1016/S0140-6736(12)61367-1

Willis, L. D., & Chandler, C. (2019). Quick fix for care, productivity, hygiene and inequality: Reframing the entrenched problem of antibiotic overuse. *BMJ Global Health*, *4*(4), e001590. https://doi.org/10.1136/bmjgh-2019-001590

6 Dueling in medical interaction

Caregivers' resistance to doctors' treatment recommendations

Introduction

In Chapters 4 and 5, I discussed the influence of caregivers and doctors on anti-biotic prescribing decisions in medical visits. I looked at caregivers' behavior in advocating for antibiotic prescriptions and doctors' behavior in delivering treatment recommendations during medical visits, respectively. These findings revealed that prescribing decisions, although seemingly within the domain of doctors' expertise, are significantly influenced by patient caregivers' treatment advocacy in medical interaction, and doctors may affect the prescribing decision by adopting an interactional style that allows for caregivers' active involvement in making prescribing decisions.

However, examining caregivers' and doctors' influence on prescribing decisions by looking at their interactional behavior separately does not fully capture the complexity and dynamics of the prescribing decision-making process. A closer examination of the sequential unfolding of the prescribing decision-making process will provide a better understanding of the relative roles of each party in the problem. If caregivers passively follow doctors' treatment recommendations, their effect on the problem of antibiotic overprescription can be considered limited. However, if caregivers take a more active role in negotiating prescribing decisions, especially when their preferred treatment does not align with the doctors' recommendations, their impact on the problem cannot be ignored. Relatedly, in the face of caregivers' resistance to treatment recommendations, if doctors more frequently pursue car-egivers' acceptance of their recommended treatment than cave in to their pressure for inappropriate prescriptions, it suggests that they may not be directly driving the antibiotic overprescription problem but rather indirectly contributing to the problem by relinquishing their role as gatekeepers of antibiotic prescriptions.

In the following sections, I will present findings about the treatment recommendation-response sequence in which doctors and patient caregivers engage in discussing the decision of antibiotics. Specifically, these findings are organized to answer the following questions: Do caregivers influence the prescribing decision by resisting doctors' treatment recommendations and initiating negotiations with their doctors? How do patient caregivers often account for their resistance to doctors' treatment recommendations? Lastly, I will examine doctors' reactions to

DOI: 10.4324/9781003243625-6

caregivers' resistance in treatment negotiation. Findings regarding whether doctors more frequently pursue caregivers' acceptance or accommodate caregivers' preferences provide crucial evidence for understanding the relative roles of doctors and patient caregivers in the antibiotic overprescription problem in China.

Background

Patient caregiver pressure and treatment decision-making interaction

The interactional behaviors that convey parental pressure for antibiotic prescription are found across different phases in medical interaction. They can occur as early as the problem presentation phase in the form of a 'candidate diagnosis' (Stivers, 2002b), in the history-taking phase through extensive detailing of particular symptoms (Stivers, 2007), in the diagnosis phase through resistance to viral diagnoses (Stivers et al., 2003a), and during the treatment recommendation phase through passive or active resistance to treatment guidance (Stivers, 2002a, 2005b). Despite their pervasive occurrence, parental pressure is more overt in the treatment recommendation phase than in any other phase. Here, the parent's view directly clashes with the doctor's view of the treatment plan for the patient. Therefore, the treatment recommendation stage is a prime location to examine how doctor–patient interaction influences prescribing decision outcomes.

Within this phase, resistance to a treatment recommendation has been found to be an important interactional resource through which parents influence prescribing outcomes. Through passive resistance (i.e., withholding of acceptance) and active resistance (e.g., questioning the doctor's treatment recommendation, proposals of alternative treatments), Stivers shows that parents actively participate in treatment decision-making and can impact prescribing decisions (Stivers, 2005b). Such communication behaviors, although widely supported as patient or parent involvement in medical decisions, can create difficulties for doctors and put them under great pressure to overprescribe.

Patient caregiver resistance, medical ideology, and the doctor–patient relationship

Beyond analyzing patient resistance as a form of interactional practice, patient resistance to treatment recommendation can also be analyzed to understand patients' orientations toward medicine and the general medical ideology – their expectations, preferences, and priorities. For instance, Bergen et al. (2018) conducted a systematic analysis of patient resistance to treatment recommendations and found that there is a cultural difference in patient orientations to prescription medicine and over-the-counter (OTC) medicine in U.S. and U.K. primary care settings. The study showed that while American patients more frequently resist OTC treatment recommendations, British patients more frequently resist prescription medicine recommendations. The distinction in patient preferences and priorities for treatment, which likely resulted from the structural differences in the two countries' healthcare systems (e.g., financing schemes, welfare policies) and their resulting medical ideology, are enacted through micro-level interactional behaviors and can be understood through detailed examinations.

Furthermore, research on patient resistance also provides important insights into patients' and doctors' orientations toward their social relationships – their entitlements and responsibilities. Beyond demonstrating that parent resistance impacts prescribing decisions, Stivers' series of studies also showed that there were normative constraints requiring parents' explicit acceptance of doctors' treatment recommendations to reach a treatment decision (Stivers, 2005b, 2005a; Stivers & Timmermans, 2020). This means that patients are no longer passive followers of doctors' treatment recommendations. A closer examination of the parents' accounts for their resistance revealed that parent resistance could pose challenges to doctors' professional authority on either or both epistemic and deontic grounds (Heritage, 2012; Stevanovic & Peräkylä, 2012; Stivers et al., 2017). Although doctors may assert and uphold their authority, such authority can also be rejected by the parents, potentially leading to a change of treatment plans (Stivers & Timmermans, 2020). This stream of research thus provides accumulating empirical evidence that the traditional paternalistic model of the doctor–patient relationship is moving toward a consumer-provider relationship in contemporary Western societies (Stivers & Timmermans, 2020).

While research in China has thus far largely pointed to organizational issues as driving inappropriate prescribing, in this paper, I investigate caregivers' responses to treatment recommendations and particularly active resistance to treatment recommendations in Chinese pediatric encounters. By focusing on caregivers' active resistance, we aim to show how Chinese caregivers influence antibiotic treatment decisions in China. Moreover, we argue that this reflects a model of the doctor–patient relationship, which underlies the interactional patterns shown in the encounters and contributes to the problem of antibiotic over-prescription in China.

Data and analytical procedures

Based on the medical interaction dataset, I investigated treatment recommendation-response sequences in a total of 187 conversations in which patients and caregivers visited for children's acute respiratory tract infection (ARTI) problems. Each conversation contains one or multiple treatment recommendations. I coded each treatment recommendation and the first turn following the treatment recommendation as its response. I excluded those treatment recommendations that contain inaudible utterances, as we cannot identify the action implemented accurately. I also excluded negatively formatted treatment recommendations and those discussions of treatment initiated by patient caregivers, as past research shows that the expected sequence trajectory is different from doctor-initiated treatment recommendations that are delivered in a positive format. In addition, I excluded contingent recommendations in which the doctors make future plans for the patient, as they do not normally lead to actual prescribing decisions in the medical visit.

In total, 573 doctor-initiated treatment recommendations and their responses were identified out of 183 medical visits (4 visits were excluded as they contain inaudible utterances in target turns). The responses were then classified into the following categories, including (1) acceptance, (2) passive resistance, and (3) active resistance. The taxonomy was based on earlier work on treatment recommendation response actions in U.K. and U.S. clinical settings (Heritage & Sefi, 1992; Stivers, 2005b); features that are specific to the Chinese language were accounted for during the coding process. I will briefly illustrate these three types of response actions in the following sections, and I will focus on caregivers' active resistance in this study.

Findings

How do caregivers respond to doctors' treatment recommendations?

Acceptance: A normatively preferred response to treatment recommendation

In making treatment decisions, doctors usually orient to the caregiver's acceptance of their treatment recommendations as relevant and expected. In an ideal case, caregivers accept doctors' treatment recommendations immediately afterward. Upon receiving the acceptance, the activity is treated as complete, and the participants move forward to the next activity. Excerpt 6.1 illustrates this.

Here, the patient is brought in for a cough. The doctor makes a treatment recommendation of cough syrup (line 1), to which the mother responds with a ready acceptance (line 2). Following the mother's explicit acceptance, the doctor starts to initiate a discussion on antipyretic (to reduce fever) as another treatment recommendation (line 3).

Excerpt 6.1 An example of caregiver's acceptance of treatment recommendation

D: Doctor
M: Mother

1	D:	吃	止咳	糖浆	不	吃	沐舒坦.	好吧?
		chi	zhike	tangjiang	bu	chi	Mushutan	haoba
		take	cough-relief	syrup	not	take	Mushutan	okay
		"Take some cough syrup, not Mushutan, OK?"						
2->	**M:**	哦	哦	哦,	好	好	好.	
		o	o	o	hao	hao	hao	
		alright	alright	alright	okay	okay	okay	
		"Alright, alright, alright. OK, OK, OK."						
3	D:	然后	退烧药	有	吧?			
		ranhou	tuishaoyao	you	ba			
		then	antipyretic	have	PRT			
		"And then, do you have antipyretics at home?"						

PRT: Particle

The excerpt shows that after receiving the mother's acceptance, the doctor treats the activity as completed and smoothly moves forward to the next activity. In addition, when the caregiver accepts the doctor's treatment recommendation, the acceptance is usually produced with no delay or hesitation – a socially preferred action in this context (Pomerantz, 1984).

Despite being socially preferred and mandated for closing the activity, acceptance is not always produced immediately following the doctor's treatment recommendations. In many cases, caregivers either *passively resist* by deferring their acceptance or *actively resist* by contesting the doctor's recommendations (Heritage & Sefi, 1992; Stivers, 2005b), and thus lead to a possible change of treatment plan. In the following, I exemplify these two types of resistance.

Passive resistance: A dispreferred response that initiates treatment negotiations

With passive resistance, the caregiver withholds acceptance by not agreeing to the proposed treatment plan. In Excerpt 6.2, the child complains about mild coughing over the past two days. The doctor diagnoses the condition as a cold with some signs of bronchitis. She thus recommends an oral treatment for the child (lines 1–2). In the face of the recommendation, the caregiver withholds her acceptance by remaining silent (line 3).

Excerpt 6.2 An example of caregiver passive resistance

D: Doctor

1	D:	感冒,	有点	气管	炎症.
		ganmao	Youdian	qiguan	yanzheng
		cold	a little	airway	inflammation
		"(He's got) a cold, a little inflammation in the airway."			
2		吃	点	药	吧?
		chi	Dian	yao	ba
		take	Some	medication	PRT
		"How about take some medicine?"			
3->		**(4.0)**	((Doctor writing on the medical records))		

PRT: Particle

Such passive withholding of acceptance (e.g., silence, unmarked acknowledgments) is hearable as resisting the doctor's treatment recommendation primarily because there is a normative orientation that caregiver acceptance is mandated for doctor's treatment recommendations (Heritage & Sefi, 1992; Stivers, 2005b). Subsequent to passive resistance, the activity usually proceeds with either the doctor's pursuit of acceptance or the caregiver's upgraded active resistance (as will be seen in Excerpt 6.3).

Active resistance: An upgraded form of dispreferred response

Apart from remaining equivocal, caregivers can be more explicit about their disagreement with the doctor's recommended treatment plan. Through active resistance, the caregiver not only withholds his or her acceptance but also makes the doctor's response relevant as a next action. Excerpt 6.3 illustrates an example of caregivers' active resistance.

Excerpt 6.3 continues on from Excerpt 6.2. In Excerpt 6.2, I showed that the doctor's oral treatment recommendation is first resisted passively by the mother with a four-second silence (line 3). Following this, the mother upgrades her passive resistance to active resistance by nominating IV antibiotic treatment for the patient (line 4). Although formulated in an interrogative format, the mother's turn postpones the acceptance of the doctor's treatment recommendation and puts the doctor under the sequential constraint of her question (Sacks et al., 1974).

Excerpt 6.3 An example of caregiver active resistance (continued from Excerpt 6.2)

M: Mother
D: Doctor

3		(4.0) ((Doctor writing on the medical records))				
4->	**M:**	不	挂水	啊?		
		bu	Guashui	a		
		no	Drip	PRT		
		"No drip?"				
5	D:	呃,	挂水	不	需要	吧,
		e	Guashui	bu	xuyao	ba
		uh	Drip	no	need	PRT
		"Uh, drip, no need for drip.				
6		先	吃	点	药.	
		xian	chi	dian	yao	
		first	Take	some	medication	
		Take some (oral) medication first.				
7		能	吃	药	好	
		neng	chi	yao	hao	
		can	Take	medication	well	
		(If he) can get well with oral medication,				
8		就	尽量	吃	药	好.
		jiu	Jinliang	chi	yao	hao
		then	Best	take	medication	well
		just try your best to take oral medication, OK?"				
9	M:	哦,	好.			
		o	hao			
		okay	OK			
		"OK, OK."				

PRT: Particle

Different from passive resistance, the caregiver's active resistance initiates a new course of action and makes relevant the doctor's response to the inquired alternative treatment (line 4). Following this active resistance, the doctor first mildly denies the need for an IV drip (line 5); she then pursues the mother's acceptance of the original treatment recommendation (oral medication) by reformulating the treatment plan as tentative (line 6) and lastly provides an explanation for her treatment rationale (lines 7–8). The activity is finally completed, with the mother displaying an explicit acceptance (line 9). It is noteworthy that although the mother agrees to the oral treatment recommendation, the doctor offers an oral antibiotic to the patient on the following, likely to be a compromise option of the inquired IV antibiotic (not shown in the excerpt).

In this section, I showed three types of responses that caregivers use in response to doctors' treatment recommendations. Table 6.1 summarizes and provides the distribution of the three types of caregiver responses.

The results show that the caregivers resist treatment recommendations and thus initiate a negotiation with their doctors about the prescribing decision, similar to their American counterparts (Stivers, 2005b). However, the proportion of active resistance is substantially higher among Chinese caregivers (31%) than among American parents (12%) (Stivers et al., 2003b). This suggests a somewhat stronger orientation by caregivers to a right to participate (or to secure antibiotics) in treatment decisions in pediatric encounters.

How do caregivers account for active resistance?

By putting the progressivity of the decision-making on hold and initiating a negotiation for an alternative treatment plan, the caregivers actively challenge doctors' medical authority. Such action is normatively dispreferred in social interaction and, thus, is often accounted for. A close examination of the grounds for their resistance

Table 6.1 Caregiver response to doctors' treatment recommendations (N = 573)

Response	Explanations	Examples	Frequency
Acceptance	Agreement with the treatment recommendation	• *OK.*	339 (59%)
Passive resistance	Withholding of acceptance	• *(2.0)*	60 (11%)
Active resistance	Contesting the treatment recommendation	• *Take oral medicine?* • *He doesn't want to take oral medicine. He'll vomit once he takes oral medicine.* • *Oral medicine doesn't work.* • *He doesn't need an IV drip?*	174 (30%)

Notes: I coded the first turn following the doctor's treatment recommendation. Therefore, although there were a number of cases in which both passive resistance and active resistance were present, I coded the cases based on whichever appeared first.

provides insights into their orientation to their role in antibiotic prescribing decisions. Based on whether the caregiver's grounds for resistance contest the doctor's epistemic authority (Heritage, 2012), I distinguish their accounts for active resistance into personal, medical, and undeclared concerns. Specifically, personal accounts are caregivers' grounds of resistance based on their personal preferences; medical accounts are caregivers' grounds of resistance based on their opinions toward the doctor's clinical judgment; undeclared concerns are when caregivers' grounds of resistance do not surface in the turn design. In the following, I show in detail how parents account for their resistance to doctors' recommendations.

Personal account for active resistance

As mentioned before, personal-based accounts for resistance involve caregivers' statements of personal preferences and real-world contingencies that make it undesirable to take the recommended treatment. While these actions pose threats to the doctor's deontic authority (Stevanovic & Peräkylä, 2012) – their ability to determine the treatment of the child – by not cooperating with the doctor's proposed action plans, they pose relatively less challenge to the doctor's epistemic authority (Heritage, 2012; Stevanovic & Peräkylä, 2012) – the doctor's knowledge of treatment – as they do not contest the doctor's clinical judgment. Excerpt 6.4 and 6.5 provide two examples of personal-based resistance.

In Excerpt 6.4, the patient is brought in for coughing. After a physical examination, the doctor finds the patient has mild airway inflammation. Reading the patient's past medical records, the doctor sees that the caregivers have a tendency to use IV infusion treatment for the patient. The doctor designs her recommendation in a way that acknowledges the caregivers' tendency to have IV infusion treatment (line 1) and then offers a recommendation of oral treatment for the patient (line 2). In such an environment, the patient's grandfather actively resists the recommendation (line 3).

Excerpt 6.4 An example of personal-based resistance: vague preference

D: Doctor
GF: Grandfather
GM: Grandmother

1	D:	你	每	次	都	挂水	啊?
		ni	mei	ci	dou	guashui	a
		you	every	time	all	drip	PRT
		"You had IV drip every time?					
2		你	吃	点	药,	怎么样	啊?
		ni	chi	dian	yao	zenmeyang	a
		you	take	some	medication	how	PRT
		How about you take some oral medication?"					

(*Continued*)

Excerpt 6.4 (Continued)

3->	**GF:**	药,	他	不	想	吃	药.
		yao	ta	bu	xiang	chi	yao
		medication	he	not	want	take	medication

"(Oral) medication, he doesn't want to take oral medication."

4	GM:	挂水.		
		guashui		
		drip		

"(He) wants to have drip."

5	D:	挂水	是	啊?
		guashui	shi	a
		drip	is	PRT

"Drip, is it?"

6	GM:	挂-	挂水	快	一点.
		gua	guashui	kuai	yidian
		drip	drip	fast	a little

"Drip, is a little faster."

7	D:	好	呢,	行	呢.
		hao	ne	xing	ne
		OK	PRT	alright	PRT

"OK. Alright.

8		那	就	给	你	挂	吧.
		na	jiu	gei	ni	gua	ba
		then	just	give	you	drip	PRT

Then (I'll) just put you on drip."

PRT: Particle

The active resistance directly challenges the doctor's deontic authority by not cooperating with the doctor on this plan of action. Consequently, it puts the progressivity of the activity on hold and prompts the doctor's further action (e.g., pursuit of acceptance of the original treatment plan, replacement with a new treatment plan) to bring the activity to closure. Although this type of resistance does not take issue with the doctor's clinical judgment, it, nonetheless, puts forward the patient's willingness as the grounds for resistance. It thus demonstrates the caregiver's understanding that (1) they have the right to participate in the treatment decisions and (2) their personal preferences are valid grounds for negotiating with the doctor.

In other cases, caregivers can be even more explicit about why they resist the treatment recommendation. Excerpt 6.5 is an example of a caregiver's active resistance that is grounded in the patient's difficulty taking the suggested medicine. In this excerpt, the main health complaint being discussed is the patient's cough. The patient is said to have coughed for over two weeks, accompanied by some sneezing and nasal congestion symptoms. After an X-ray and blood tests, the doctor finds no clear signs of *Mycoplasma pneumoniae*. She then recommends oral antibiotic treatment for the patient (lines 2–4). This oral treatment recommendation is resisted by the mother (lines 5–7) and the grandmother (lines 9–10, lines 12–14) by citing the child's difficulty in taking oral medicine.

Excerpt 6.5 An example of personal-based resistance: difficulty in taking medicine

D: Doctor
M: Mother
GM: Grandmother

1		((A few lines of blood test results discussion omitted))						
2	D:	你	就算	要是	没	口服	过	药,
		ni	jiusuan	yaoshi	mei	koufu	guo	yao
		you	even	if	not	oral	ASP	medicine

"Even if you haven't taken any oral medicine yet,

3		你	给	他	吃	点	那个	阿奇霉素
		ni	gei	ta	chi	dian	nage	aqimeisu
		you	give	him	take	some	that	*Azithromycin*

you can give him some oral azithromycin take.

4		也	行,	口服.
		ye	xing	koufu
		also	fine	oral

It would also do. Oral medication."

5->	**M:**	我	家里	吧,	口服	药	全	有,
		wo	jiali	ba	koufu	yao	quan	you
		My	home	PRT	oral	medicine	all	have

"I have all those oral medicine at home.

6->		[然后	他	不	吃:,
		ranhou	ta	bu	chi
		then	he	not	take

and he doesn't take it.

7->		一	吃	完	就	吐.
		yi	chi	wan	jiu	tu
		once	take	up	then	vomit

He'll vomit once he finishes taking the oral medicine."

8	D:	[但	他	吃	不	进去,
		dan	ta	chi	bu	jinqu
		but	he	take	not	in

"But he can't take it in."

9->	GM:	他	一	吃	完	就	吐,
		ta	yi	chi	wan	jiu	tu
		he	once	take	up	then	vomit

"He'll vomit once he finishes taking the oral medicine.

10->		哎呀,	吐	那	到处	都	是.
		aiya	tu	na	daochu	dou	shi
		alas	vomit	there	everywhere	all	is

Alas. He vomited everywhere."

11	D:	那	你	吐	完	再	喂	呢?
		na	ni	tu	wan	zai	wei	ne
		then	you	vomit	over	again	feed	PRT

"Then what about you feed him again after he finishes vomiting?"

12->	GM:	再	喂	也	不	行,
		zai	wei	ye	bu	xing
		again	feed	also	not	alright

Excerpt 6.5 (Continued)

		"Feeding him again won't work.						
13->		不	吃	了	那	就,	也	不
		bu	chi	le	na	jiu	ye	bu
		not	take	PRT	that	then	also	not
		He won't take it then, won't take it again.						
14->		我	喂	也	喂	不	进去.	
		wo	wei	ye	wei	bu	jinqu	
		I	feed	also	feed	not	in	
		I can't feed it in, even if I feed him again."						
15	D:	那	你	就	输	点	滴流,	要不-
		na	ni	jiu	shu	dian	diliu	yaobu
		then	you	then	give	some	drip	otherwise
		"Then you just have some IV drip, otherwise."						
16	M:	打	两	天	滴流	呗.		
		da	liang	tian	diliu	bei		
		have	two	day	drip	PRT		
		"Have two-days' drip."						

PRT: Particle

As shown in the excerpt, upon receiving the doctor's oral antibiotic treatment recommendation, the caregivers actively resist it by presenting the child's difficulty in taking oral medicine. This concern, presented as coming from the caregivers' personal experiences, does not take issue with the doctor's clinical judgment of the patient's condition or the efficacy of the suggested treatment. Instead, it puts on the table a real-world contingency of the patient. In the face of such resistance, although the doctor pursues the caregivers' acceptance by suggesting this difficulty may be overcome by repeated efforts (line 11), this pursuit fails, and the doctor thus concedes with an offer of IV treatment (line 15). Again, the caregiver's use of a personal-based account for their resistance displays that they orient to their rights in participating in the treatment decision and their personal experience or preference as equally entitled to be considered in decision-making.

Medical-based account for active resistance

A second account that caregivers offer for resistance is medical-based. As mentioned earlier, through active resistance, caregivers question the recommended treatment or even propose an alternative treatment. In contrast to personal-based accounts, resistance that is grounded in medical-related accounts contests the doctor's medical judgment, thus posing a greater challenge to the doctor's medical authority. At its most extreme, by proposing alternative treatment, caregivers directly counter the doctor's clinical judgment. Excerpt 6.6 illustrates questioning the recommended treatment; Excerpt 6.7 shows a caregiver proposing alternative treatment.

In Excerpt 6.6, the child is visiting for a fever. Before visiting the doctor, the caregiver had already put the child on oral medication. Finding no signs of bacterial infection, the doctor suggests the patient continue to use the oral medication (lines 1–2). After a micropause at line 3, the doctor begins to expand her oral treatment recommendation, referencing the blood test result (line 4) to likely further account for why she is recommending oral medication. However, this is overlapped with the caregiver's active resistance at line 5.

Excerpt 6.6 An example of medical-related resistance: questioning the treatment

D: Doctor
GM1: Grandmother

1	D:	实际上	啊,	你	这个				
		shijishang	a	ni	zhege				
		actually	PRT	you	this				
		"Actually, with this (blood test result),							
2		还	要	继续	吃	药.			
		hai	yao	jixu	chi	yao			
		still	need	continue	take	medication			
		you still need to go on taking (oral) medication."							
3		(.)							
4		[你	这个	血象	啊-				
		ni	zhege	xuexiang	a				
		you	this	hemogram	PRT				
		"Your hemogram-"							
5>	**GM1:**	[没的	用	哎,					
		meide	yong	ai					
		no	use	PRT					
		"It won't work."							
6	D:	你	这个	血象	也	不	高	哎,	
		ni	zhege	xuexiang	ye	bu	gao	ai	
		you	this	hemogram	also	not	high	PRT	
		"Your hemogram (value) isn't high."							

PRT: Particle

The active resistance is designed as a negative evaluation of the treatment, assessing the treatment as ineffective. This action challenges at least two aspects of the doctor's medical authority: first, it challenges the doctor's deontic authority (Stevanovic & Peräkylä, 2012) by not undertaking to follow the doctor's proposed plan of action. Second, it further contests the doctor's epistemic authority by denying the medical appropriateness of the treatment – *It won't work*. Following the resistance, the doctor justifies her recommendation by citing the blood test results as clinical evidence again (line 6). Thus, it registers the doctor's understanding that the caregiver's resistance is challenging her clinical judgment.

Excerpt 6.7 shows a case of medical-based active resistance taking the form of a counterproposal of treatment. The excerpt is the same as Excerpts 6.2 and 6.3. As mentioned earlier, the doctor recommends that the patient take oral medication for his cold and mild bronchitis. In the face of the oral treatment recommendation, the mother actively resists it by making a counterproposal of IV infusion treatment at line 4.

Excerpt 6.7 An example of medical-based resistance: counterproposal

D: Doctor
M: Mother

1	D:	感冒,	有点	气管	炎症.				
		ganmao	youdian	qiguan	yanzheng				
		cold	a little	airway	inflammation				
		"(He's got) a cold, a little inflammation in the airway.							
2		吃	点	药	吧?				
		chi	dian	yao	ba				
		take	some	medication	PRT				
		Take some oral medication, OK?"							
3		(4.0)							
4>	**M:**	不	挂水	啊?					
		bu	guashui	a					
		no	drip	PRT					
		"No drip?"							
5	D:	呃,	挂水	不	需要	吧,			
		e	guashui	bu	xuyao	ba			
		uh	drip	no	need	PRT			
		"Uh, drip, no need for drip.							
6		先	吃	点	药.	能	吃	药	好
		xian	chi	dian	yao	neng	chi	yao	hao
		first	take	some	medication	can	take	medication	well
		Take some (oral) medication first. (If he) can get well with oral medication,							
7		就	尽量	吃	药	好.			
		jiu	jinliang	chi	yao	hao			
		then	best	take	medication	well			
		Then just try your best to take oral medication, OK?"							

PRT: Particle

The mother does not in any way affiliate with the doctor's proposed treatment, but she goes beyond this. Her active resistance queries an alternative treatment plan (IV antibiotics), which orients to the doctor's treatment recommendation as inferior to the mother's own treatment proposal. Although the mother's interrogatively designed request for confirmation treats the doctor as at least nominally deciding, her query is, nonetheless, hearable as proposing IV antibiotics. In doing so, her action challenges the doctor's epistemic authority in that it takes issue with the doctor's clinical judgment.

The doctor's response displays that she is under pressure from the caregiver. This can be evidenced by the fact that (1) she prefaces her turn with *e* ("uh"), marking her denial of the mother's proposal as dispreferred (Pomerantz, 1984); (2) in line 5, she denies the mother's proposal with a turn produced with a final partial *ba*, creating a sense of proposal to be approved by the mother (Li & Thompson, 1981); and (3) although the doctor pursues the mother's acceptance of the original treatment recommendation, she reformulates the recommendation as a tentative arrangement that is subject to further change.

In sum, caregivers' medical-related active resistance displays an orientation toward their rights and entitlement to participate in their children's treatment decision-making. In addition, it also shows that their knowledge or experience is on par with that of doctors, which poses significant challenges to the medical authority of doctors. In response, doctors also demonstrate an orientation to caregivers' rights to participate in treatment decisions; however, they, nevertheless, display themselves as under substantial pressure from the caregivers and thereby frequently justify their treatment recommendations with elaborations of their clinical judgment.

Undeclared basis for active resistance

While in some cases caregivers resist doctors' treatment recommendations on the basis of personal or medical concerns, they sometimes actively resist doctors' treatment recommendations with question-intoned partial repeats or open-class initiators (Drew, 1997) that clearly indicate resistance but not the basis of that resistance. Still, they problematize the previous treatment recommendation and make relevant a response from the doctor through their turn designs (Schegloff, 2007). In the face of this class of resistance, although doctors have the flexibility to treat it as either a hearing problem or an understanding problem, I find that they more frequently treat it as a medical concern for acceptance. Excerpt 6.8 provides an illustration.

In this excerpt, the patient is brought in for a cough and sore throat. Before visiting the doctor, the caregiver has already given the child Dalifen *(cefixime)* – an oral antibiotic. Since the physical examination finds no sign of bacterial infection (prior to the excerpt shown), the doctor recommends non-antibiotic oral treatment for the patient (line 1). In the face of this recommendation, the mother actively resists it by producing a question-intoned partial repeat of the doctor's treatment recommendation (line 2) and makes relevant a doctor's response on the next.

Excerpt 6.8 An example of undeclared basis for resistance

D: Doctor
M: Mother

1	D:	你:,	吃	点	药	吧.		
		ni	chi	dian	yao	ba		
		you	take	some	medicine	PRT		
		"You, how about you take some oral medicine?"						
2->	**M:**	吃	点	药	啊?			
		chi	dian	yao	a			
		take	some	medicine	PRT			
		"Take some oral medicine?"						
3	D:	哎,	你	前面	达力芬	其实	刚	开始
		ai	ni	qianmian	Dalifen	qishi	gang	kaishi
		yeah	you	before	Dalifen	actually	just	beginning
		"Yeah, actually you don't have to take Dalifen before,						

(Continued)

Excerpt 6.8 (Continued)

4	倒	不	要	吃.
	dao	bu	yao	chi
	contrary	not	need	take
	at the very beginning."			

PRT: Particle

Following the mother's active resistance, the doctor first confirms the treatment recommendation with *ai* ("yeah") at line 3 and then goes on to justify her treatment recommendation by denying the necessity and appropriateness of the caregiver using Dalifen (an oral antibiotic) before the medical visit (lines 3–4).

Going through the dataset, I find that doctors respond to this class of active resistance with medical-related justifications most frequently in 61% of the cases; simple confirmation occurs in 35% of cases; in the remaining 4% of cases, the doctor elaborates with non-medical concerns to pursue caregiver's acceptance. Thus, even when the caregiver does not articulate the grounds for their active resistance, the doctor frequently orients to them as having medical-related concerns and thus pursues their acceptance accordingly.

In sum, these three types of caregiver active resistance all pose a challenge to a doctor's deontic authority by not undertaking the doctor's proposed treatment plans (Stevanovic & Peräkylä, 2012; Stivers, 2005b; Stivers & Timmermans, 2020). Furthermore, the three types of active resistance also pose varying degrees of challenge to the doctor's epistemic authority. Medical-based active resistance poses the highest degree of challenge to the doctor's epistemic authority, as the caregiver trespasses into the doctor's domain of professional knowledge by contesting the medical appropriateness of the treatment recommendation. Personal-related resistance, on the other hand, poses a lower degree of challenge to the doctor's epistemic authority, as caregivers do not contest the clinical judgment of the doctor's treatment plan but put forward their own desires or preferences as the grounds for resistance. However, preference-based resistance can be treated by doctors as the most problematic basis for resistance, as it also may pit caregivers against clinicians in terms of whose judgment should prevail (Stivers & Timmermans, 2020). Lastly, with the unsurfaced concern resistance, although caregivers do not explicitly challenge the doctor on either personal or medical grounds, they are mostly oriented by doctors as challenging the medical grounds and thus are usually justified with medical-related elaborations.

Distribution of caregivers' accounts for active resistance

Due to doctors' medical authority, one would expect medical-based active resistance to be used less frequently by caregivers than personal-based active resistance. However, I find the opposite. Table 6.2 shows the relative distribution of the three types of accounts for active resistance across the dataset.

Table 6.2 Caregivers' accounts for active resistance (N=174)

Type of accounts	Frequency	Percentage
Personal-related	11	6%
Undeclared basis	77	45%
Medical-related	86	49%
Total	**174**	**100%**

As shown in the table, despite the fact that caregivers' medical-based resistance poses a higher level of challenge to doctors' medical authority than personal-based resistance because it contests both their deontic and epistemic authority, it is, nonetheless, the most frequently used. Moreover, even when caregivers' active resistance does not surface their grounds for resistance as either medical- or personal-related, doctors tend to treat them as medically related and thus are more likely to perceive challenges to their authority and pressure for inappropriate prescribing. Finally, if we return to Extract 6.4, note that although the grandfather and grandmother both begin with personal-based resistance, the grandmother shifts to medical-based grounds when she states that the drip works faster. Thus, although caregivers accept doctors' recommendations most of the time, when they resist, they most commonly do so in a way that challenges the doctor's authority, and both doctors and caregivers orient to caregivers as seeking to determine treatment for their children.

How do doctors react to caregivers' active resistance?

Given that caregivers are oriented to having the right to contest doctors' medical authority, how do doctors respond when their medical authority is being challenged? In this section, I argue that although doctors strive to uphold their medical judgment, they, nonetheless, succumb to caregiver pressure from time to time. In the following, I first show the relative distribution of doctors' reactions to caregivers' active resistance; I then use two examples to illustrate how caregivers' active resistance and doctors' reactions unfold in conversation.

Distribution of doctors' reactions

On the one hand, this study finds that in a majority of cases, caregivers ultimately accept doctors' recommendations, seeming to suggest that doctors in China retain strong medical authority. Yet, I also find that caregivers resist more frequently than in the U.S. pediatric context, displaying an orientation to having strong rights to dictate treatment. These conflicting findings lead to the question of how doctors react to caregiver resistance. In Table 6.3, I show the influence that caregivers' active resistance has on treatment decisions.

The results indicate that even when caregivers actively resist treatment recommendations, doctors strive to uphold their original treatment plans. Across the 174 active resistance cases, they change their treatment plans 18% of the time

Table 6.3 Doctors' reaction to caregivers' active resistance (N=174)

Status of treatment plan	Frequency	Percentage
Change of treatment plan	31	18%
No change of treatment plan	143	82%
Total	**174**	**100%**

and maintain their original plan 82% of the time. When we consider that nearly 1 out of every 5 visits result in a change, nearly always to a more advanced form of antibiotic prescription (e.g., IV rather than oral), this reflects that caregivers are having a substantial influence on prescribing outcomes. This takes on even more significance when we consider that this is *only* the influence that caregivers exert through *active resistance* (e.g., see other means to influence prescribing in Stivers and Timmermans (2021)). In what follows, I show how doctors fail and manage to uphold their treatment plans in particular cases.

Doctor concession to caregiver pressure

Excerpt 6.9 involves caregivers' active resistance leading to a change of treatment plan. This is a continuation of Excerpt 6.6. As described earlier, the patient's condition is diagnosed as a viral infection; the doctor suggests the patient take oral medication as the treatment plan. However, the caregiver actively resists the treatment recommendation by calling into question the efficacy of the suggested oral treatment (line 5) (Bergen et al., 2018).

Excerpt 6.9 An example of doctor's change of treatment plan (continued from Excerpt 6.6)

GM1: Grandmother1
D: Doctor
GM2: Grandmother2

5	GM1:	[没的	用	哎,				
		meide	yong	ai				
		no	use	PRT				
		"It won't work."						
6	D:	你	这个	血象	也	不	高	哎,
		ni	zhege	xuexiang	ye	bu	gao	ai
		you	this	hemogram	also	not	high	PRT
		"Your hemogram (value) isn't high."						
7	GM2:	不	高	是	啊?=			
		bu	gao	shi	a			

(Continued)

Excerpt 6.9 (Continued)

		not	high	is		PRT		
		"Not high, is it?"						
8	D:	嗯,	才	五千		多.		
		en	cai	wuqian		duo		
		yeah	only	five-thousand		over		
		"Yeah, it's just over five-thousand."						
9	GM1:	哎,	对的	哎,				
		ai	duide	ai				
		yeah	right	PRT				
		"Yeah, right.						
10		我家	吃	药	吃	不	住	哎.
		wojia	chi	yao	chi	bu	zhu	ai
		ours	take	medicine	take	not	down	PRT
		Oral medicine can't bring it down for us."						
11	GM2:	挂	两	天	水-			
		gua	liang	tian	shui			
		drip	two	day	drip			
		"Have two-days' drip."						
12->	**D:**	你	挂	两	天	水,		
		ni	gua	liang	tian	shui		
		you	drip	two	day	drip		
		"You have two-days' drip.						
13->		挂	那个-	抗病毒的,				
		gua	nage	kangbingdude				
		drip	that	anti-viral				
		Use that anti-viral medicine for drip.						
14->		你	挂	那个	头孢	实际上	也	没用.
		ni	gua	nage	toubao	shijishang	ye	meiyong
		you	drip	that	Cephlo	actually	also	useless
		(If) you use Cephalo for drip, it doesn't really help."						

PRT: Particle

As shown in the excerpt, following the caregiver's resistance, the doctor pursues the caregiver's acceptance by citing the blood test results (lines 6, 8). Although the caregiver acknowledges the doctor's information and her evaluation that the result is not problematic (line 9), the caregiver (GM1) still resists the oral treatment recommendation by denying its efficacy (line 10). In addition, the other accompanying caregiver (GM2) further upgrades the active resistance by nominating an alternative treatment – IV infusion treatment (line 11).

Subsequent to repeated active resistance, the doctor succumbs to the caregivers' pressure and switches to provide an IV infusion treatment to the patient instead (lines 12–14). It is noteworthy that although the doctor agrees to change her treatment recommendation, the change only accommodates the caregivers' preference in terms of treatment *modality* (from oral treatment to IV infusion) but not their preferred antibiotic (Cephalo). This shows that even in compromised cases, the doctor still strives hard to retain her professional authority.

Doctor withstanding caregiver pressure

Excerpt 6.10 illustrates an example of the doctor's pursuit of acceptance following the caregiver's active resistance, which succeeds in getting the caregiver on board. The excerpt is continued from Excerpt 6.7. In this case, although the mother directly challenges the doctor on both deontic and epistemic grounds by making a counterproposal to the doctor's treatment recommendation, the doctor actively pursues the mother's acceptance of the original treatment plan, with which the mother then agrees (line 8).

Excerpt 6.10 An example of doctor's pursuit of acceptance (continued from Excerpt 6.3)

M: Mother
D: Doctor

4	M:	不	挂水	啊?				
		bu	guashui	a				
		no	drip	PRT				
		"No drip?"						
5>	**D:**	呃,	挂水	不	需要	吧,		
		e	guashui	bu	xuyao	ba		
		uh	drip	no	need	PRT		
		"Uh, no need for drip.						
6>		先	吃	点	药.	能	吃	药	好
		xian	chi	dian	yao	neng	chi	yao	hao
		first	take	some	medication	can	take	medication	well
		Take some (oral) medication first. (If he) can get well with oral medication,						
7>		就	尽量	吃	药	好.		
		jiu	jinliang	chi	yao	hao		
		then	best	take	medication	well		
		just try the best to take oral medication, OK?"						
8	M:	哦,	好.					
		o	hao					
		okay	OK					
		" OK, OK."						

PRT: Particle

As shown in the excerpt, the doctor actively pursues the mother's acceptance of the original treatment plan (lines 5–7). The pursuit of acceptance directly addresses the mother's active resistance by providing the rationale for the treatment plan – oral treatment is preferred over IV infusion treatment and thus is chosen as a better plan for the patient's current condition. In addition, it is worth noticing that while the doctor refuses to accommodate the mother's preference, she acknowledges her preference by formulating the treatment plan as tentative, which opens up a future possibility of using the IV infusion treatment if the patient's condition gets worse.

In the previous sections, I have shown that through active resistance, the caregivers purposefully involve themselves in the decision-making process of their children's treatment plans. By putting the activity progressivity on hold and by challenging the doctor on either or both epistemic grounds and deontic grounds, caregivers prompt doctors to react to their active resistance – whether this leads to them withstanding and pursuing the caregiver's acceptance or to conceding and changing the original treatment plan.

Taken together, the quantitative and qualitative analyses of caregivers' active resistance and doctors' responses reveal two points. First, the caregivers' active resistance places the doctors under pressure to yield their professional judgments. As seen from Excerpt 6.9, although the doctors do not believe it is appropriate to prescribe antibiotic treatment, they may still prescribe it under such pressure. Yielding even 18% of the time leads to a significant escalation of inappropriate prescribing for viral illnesses. Second, although caregivers display high levels of entitlement to influence treatment decisions, doctors still strive to preserve their professional authority, which is essential for gatekeeping prescription medicine such as antibiotics.

Conclusion

In this chapter, rather than focusing on doctors' behavior or caregivers' behaviors separately, I examined the sequential unfolding of the treatment recommendation-response sequences between doctors and caregivers in medical interaction. The findings showed that in treatment decision interaction, while Chinese caregivers express their personal preferences for treatment similarly to their American counterparts (Stivers & Timmermans, 2020), they more commonly orient themselves as on par with their doctors to decide the best course of treatment for the patient. It, thus, poses threats to the doctors' epistemic primacy in making clinical judgments and deontic authority in deciding on a treatment plan.

In addition, through analyzing caregivers' responses to doctors' treatment recommendations, I showed that despite their prescription medicine status, antibiotics are considered by caregivers as commodities that are negotiable with their doctors. Caregivers actively influence treatment decisions by resisting doctors' non-antibiotic treatment recommendations, which is similar to their American counterparts (Stivers, 2002a, 2005b). However, different from American parents, Chinese caregivers more commonly engage in negotiations with their doctors on infusion antibiotics versus oral antibiotics. In other words, while there is a medical ideology among American parents that favors prescription medicine over over-the-counter (OTC) medicine (Bergen et al., 2018), among Chinese caregivers, there is an additional preference for infusion antibiotics over oral antibiotics. In such a prescribing culture, doctors are exposed to greater pressure for overprescribing, and oral antibiotics may be prescribed as a compromise option for infusion antibiotics.

These findings revealed that the model of the doctor–patient relationship that we see in this study is somewhat distinct from that in Western societies. Although research provides growing evidence that medical authority is declining and the doctor–patient relationship is gradually moving away from a paternalistic model (Light, 2010; Peräkylä, 2006; Starr, 1982; Stivers & Timmermans, 2020), doctors are still generally considered to have a high level of cultural and social authorities in Western societies (but see Ostermann (2021)). However, in the Chinese pediatric setting, we see that while doctors work hard to retain their authority, their authority is consistently challenged by patient caregivers. Patient caregivers appear to be nudging the doctor–patient relationship closer to a consumerist model.

The model of the doctor–patient relationship and degree of medical authority is consequential for health outcomes. In the case of antibiotic prescribing, although antibiotics are supposed to be prescribed based on the doctor's clinical judgment, caregivers in the Chinese clinical setting often orient themselves as entitled consumers and present their personal preferences, experience, or popular ideologies as equally legitimate bases for participating in treatment decisions, with doctors' professional expertise. This model of the doctor–patient relationship reflected in the Chinese pediatric setting nowadays is thus consequential on the antibiotic over-prescription problem, as it renders the doctors powerless to gatekeep prescription medicine when patients/caregivers demand.

References

Bergen, C., Stivers, T., Barnes, R. K., Heritage, J., McCabe, R., Thompson, L., & Toerien, M. (2018). Closing the deal: A cross-cultural comparison of treatment resistance. *Health Communication*, *33*(11), 1377–1388. https://doi.org/10.1080/10410236.2017.1350917

Drew, P. (1997). "Open" class repair initiators in response to sequential sources of troubles in conversation. *Journal of Pragmatics*, *28*(1), 69–101. https://doi.org/10.1016/S0378-2166(97)89759-7

Heritage, J. (2012). The epistemic engine: Sequence organization and territories of knowledge. *Research on Language and Social Interaction*, *45*(1), 30–52. https://doi.org/10.1080/08351813.2012.646685

Heritage, J., & Sefi, S. (1992). Dilemmas of advice: Aspects of the delivery and reception of advice in interactions between health visitors and first time mothers. In *Talk at Work* (pp. 3–65). Cambridge University Press.

Li, C. N., & Thompson, S. A. (1981). *Mandarin Chinese: A functional reference grammar*. University of California Press.

Light, D. W. (2010). Health-care professions, markets, and countervailing powers. In *Handbook of medical sociology* (6th ed., pp. 270–289). Vanderbilt University Press.

Ostermann, A. C. (2021). Women's (limited) agency over their sexual bodies: Contesting contraceptive recommendations in Brazil. *Social Science & Medicine*, *290*, 114276. https://doi.org/10.1016/j.socscimed.2021.114276

Peräkylä, A. (2006). Communicating and responding to diagnosis. In *Communication in medical care: Interaction between primary care physicians and patients*. Cambridge University Press.

Pomerantz, A. (1984). *Agreeing and disagreeing with assessments: Some features of preferred/dispreferred turn shaped*. Communication Faculty Scholarship. http://scholarsarchive.library.albany.edu/cas_communication_scholar/3

Sacks, H., Schegloff, E., & Jefferson, G. (1974). A simplest systematics for the organization of turn-taking for conversation. *Language*, *50*, 696–735.

Schegloff, E. (2007). *Sequence organization in interaction: A primer in conversation analysis*. Cambridge University Press.

Starr, P. (1982). *The social transformation of American medicine: The rise of a sovereign profession and the making of a vast industry*. Basic Books.

Stevanovic, M., & Peräkylä, A. (2012). Deontic authority in interaction: The right to announce, propose, and decide. *Research on Language & Social Interaction, 45*(3), 297–321. https://doi.org/10.1080/08351813.2012.699260

Stivers, T. (2002a). Participating in decisions about treatment: Overt parent pressure for antibiotic medication in pediatric encounters. *Social Science & Medicine, 54*(7), 1111–1130.

Stivers, T. (2002b). "Symptoms only" and "candidate diagnoses": Presenting the problem in pediatric encounters. *Health Communication, 3*(14), 299–338.

Stivers, T. (2005a). Non-antibiotic treatment recommendations: Delivery formats and implications for parent resistance. *Social Science & Medicine, 5*(60), 949–964.

Stivers, T. (2005b). Parent resistance to physicians' treatment recommendations: One resource for initiating a negotiation of the treatment decision. *Health Communication, 181*(1), 41–74.

Stivers, T. (2007). *Prescribing under pressure: Physician-parent conversations and antibiotics*. Oxford University Press.

Stivers, T., Heritage, J., Barnes, R. K., McCabe, R., Thompson, L., & Toerien, M. (2017). Treatment recommendations as actions. *Health Communication*, 1–10. https://doi.org/10.1080/10410236.2017.1350913

Stivers, T., Mangione-Smith, R., Elliott, M. N., McDonald, L., & Heritage, J. (2003a). Why do physicians think parents expect antibiotics? What parents report vs what physicians believe. *The Journal of Family Practice, 52*(2), 140–147.

Stivers, T., Mangione-Smith, R., Elliott, M. N., McDonald, L., & Heritage, J. (2003b). Why do physicians think parents expect antibiotics? What parents report vs what physicians believe. *The Journal of Family Practice, 52*(2), 140–148.

Stivers, T., & Timmermans, S. (2020). Medical authority under siege: How clinicians transform patient resistance into acceptance. *Journal of Health and Social Behavior, 61*(1), 60–78. https://doi.org/10.1177/0022146520902740

Stivers, T., & Timmermans, S. (2021). Arriving at no: Patient pressure to prescribe antibiotics and physicians' responses. *Social Science & Medicine, 290*, 114007. https://doi.org/10.1016/j.socscimed.2021.114007

7 Conclusion

At the high-level panel on World Health Day 2011, Margaret Chan, the WHO Director-General, delivered an important speech titled "Combat antimicrobial resistance conference: No action today, no cure tomorrow." She not only highlighted the stark reality the world is facing but also emphasized that our behaviors are largely responsible for this situation. Despite this loud and clear message, the situation has not changed significantly, especially in countries and regions with rapid economic development and increased access to antibiotics. China also faces this problem. As one of the largest manufacturers and consumers of antibiotics in the world, its problem is concerning and requires urgent attention. This book aims to enhance our understanding of the problem by presenting a perspective that is often overlooked and proposing actions that can be implemented in daily medical encounters.

In the following sections, I will first summarize the main findings of each empirical chapter. This will be followed by a discussion of action proposals to reduce antibiotic overprescription in Chinese pediatric primary care settings. Lastly, I will conclude the book with three core messages as the implications for this study.

A summary of chapter findings

Chapter 2 examined the macro-level historical and institutional factors of the antibiotic overprescription problem. Besides contextualizing the findings of the book by describing a typical medical visit in Chinese pediatric care and introducing the organization of the healthcare system, I argued that the various structural issues related to the organization of the healthcare system contributed to the antibiotic overprescription problem by creating a complex matrix of perverse incentives for doctors' overprescription. These perverse incentives, despite being removed in later reforms, still cast an indirect form of influence by creating an antibiotic-saturated medical culture and shaping patients' and caregivers' behaviors and attitudes related to antibiotics.

Chapter 3 examined patient caregivers' use and desire for antibiotics before medical visits and their relationship with the prescribed medications in medical visits. When children showed symptoms of the common cold, many caregivers used non-prescribed antibiotics. If self-management failed, caregivers would take their child to a medical visit, often expecting stronger treatment, such as antibiotic

DOI: 10.4324/9781003243625-7

intravenous infusions. Statistical evidence shows that caregivers who used non-prescribed antibiotics before a medical visit and had a desire for antibiotic prescriptions were more likely to receive antibiotic prescriptions from their doctors during the visit. These findings suggest that even before doctors and caregivers meet in a clinical encounter, the effect of caregivers' behaviors and attitudes on antibiotic prescription is already taking shape.

Chapter 4 investigated the interactional practices that patient caregivers often used and were subject to doctors' understanding as advocating for antibiotic prescriptions in medical encounters. The findings showed that these advocating practices were frequently used, occurring in more than half of the cases in the dataset. When caregivers used one or more of these practices, the likelihood of doctors prescribing antibiotics increased by 9–14 times. Furthermore, a cross-cultural comparison of the findings in Chinese and American pediatric settings revealed that although caregivers in both countries used these practices, Chinese caregivers used them much more frequently and tended to use more overt forms of advocacy. It, thus, suggests that patient caregivers actively influence prescribing decisions and put doctors under great pressure to prescribe inappropriately.

Chapter 5 examined the role of doctors in prescribing decisions by analyzing their treatment recommendations in medical encounters. The findings indicate that, first, doctors did not prescribe antibiotics to their patients as frequently as expected based on the popular supply-side theory. Second, doctors did not use a dominant conversational style to deliver treatment recommendations and, thus, did not coerce caregivers into accepting their recommendations. These results suggest that doctors consider caregiver involvement to be relevant, if not more important, in prescribing decisions, even though treatment recommendations are traditionally viewed as within the doctors' domain of expertise. Consequently, doctors may no longer actively drive the problem of antibiotic overprescription nowadays; instead, they may contribute to the problem passively by conceding to caregivers' pressure. The nature of the doctor-caregiver relationship plays a significant role in shaping their interaction, which, in turn, affects the outcome of prescribing decisions.

In Chapter 6, I analyzed the relative roles of doctors and patient caregivers in prescribing decisions by examining the sequential unfolding of treatment recommendation-response sequences in medical interactions. The findings revealed that caregivers were not passive followers of doctors' treatment recommendations. On the contrary, they actively influenced treatment decisions by resisting doctors' recommendations and initiating negotiations for desirable treatments. Caregivers' resistance, which occurred quite frequently in the dataset, indicated that they regarded their opinions as on par with those of the doctors in the prescribing decision. In most cases, doctors pursued caregivers' acceptance of their original recommendations, but they did not always succeed. These findings suggested that prescribing decisions were not made by doctors alone but were negotiated between doctors and caregivers.

Taking stock, these findings reveal that antibiotic overprescription in China should not be understood as solely attributed to doctors' financial incentives or patients' irrational demands. Instead, it should be understood as a social and interactional process between doctors and patient caregivers, which involves complexities at both micro-level and macro-level. These complexities primarily encompass the following three aspects.

First, patients are no longer passive followers of their doctors' treatment recommendations, as suggested by the *sick role theory* in a paternalistic model of the doctor–patient relationship (Parsons, 1951). Instead, patients and caregivers actively bring in their experiences, knowledge, and opinions to the decision-making process. Doctors cannot force their patients to agree with their judgments, nor can they coerce them into accepting their treatment recommendations based on their professional authority. Therefore, the evolving nature of the doctor–patient relationship contributes to the problem.

Second, the complexities of human social interaction also contribute to the problem. As demonstrated in this book, explicit requests for antibiotics from caregivers (*e.g., Doctor, please prescribe me some antibiotics.*) are relatively uncommon. More frequently, overprescription is influenced by implicit interactional practices that convey pressure (*e.g., inquiries or partial repeats*). Research has shown that these practices do not always stem from caregivers' actual demands for antibiotics but rather demands for knowledge (Cabral et al., 2019; Stivers et al., 2003). In a time-pressured setting, doctors may misinterpret or simply determine these implicit interactional practices as demands for antibiotics. As a result, antibiotics are prescribed in order to avoid prolonged communication.

Third, the micro-level details of doctor-caregiver interaction are not isolated from but, rather, intertwined with the historical transformation, institutional arrangements, and cultural factors at the macro-level. The commodification of the healthcare services, brought by the historical and social changes of the country, profoundly impacts how doctors practice medicine, how the general public understand medicine and seek care, and how doctors and patients orient toward their rights and incumbency within their social relationship.

Given these findings, the next relevant question is: What can we do to reduce inappropriate antibiotic prescribing? Perhaps lessons can be learned from reviewing intervention programs that have been found effective in similar contexts and identifying practices with similar potentials.

On the following, I will first briefly review DART – Dialogue Around Respiratory Illness Treatment – one of the most successful intervention programs conducted in U.S. pediatric settings to reduce inappropriate antibiotic prescribing; I will then review findings of two conversation analytical studies and discuss the potential communication opportunities they have for doctors to address patient caregiver pressure and create teachable moments in Chinese pediatric settings.

Training doctors essential communication skills

The DART program: experience from U.S. pediatrics

The DART intervention trial was a cluster-randomized, stepped-wedge, clinical trial that allowed enrolled clinicians, including pediatricians and pediatric nurse practitioners, to receive the intervention across 19 American primary care pediatric practices between 2015 and 2018. Physicians were provided with a three-module training program including (1) a 25-minute online tutorial on evidence-based communication strategies and antibiotic prescribing, (2) a 40-minute webinar, and (3) three booster video-vignette sessions to recap best communication practices and test clinicians' understanding (*Dialogue Around Respiratory Illness Treatment (DART)*, 2016; Mangione-Smith et al., 2022). The results showed that, among 72,723 acute respiratory tract infections (ARTIs) visits by 29,762 patients, the DART program intervention trial decreased overall antibiotic prescribing for ARTIs by 7% and inappropriate antibiotic prescribing for ARTIs by 40% (Mangione-Smith et al., 2022).

One of the program's core features is that its intervention strategies and training content are evidence-based. Two communication behaviors that are identified in conversation analysis study and found significantly impact the prescribing outcomes are highlighted in the DART program:

Communication behavior 1: *Delivering a combined, two-part treatment recommendation that includes both a negative recommendation and a positive recommendation.*

Negative recommendation is a method of delivering treatment recommendation that aims to rule out the need for antibiotics. For example, a doctor might say, "What we have here is a really bad cold, so nothing an antibiotic will help." *Positive recommendation* is a method of delivering treatment recommendation in which the doctor suggests actions that parents can take to reduce their child's symptoms. For instance, they might advise, "Giving her an extra pillow at night can help with draining the congestion." These two delivery practices were initially identified in a conversation analysis (CA) study of physicians' treatment recommendation actions using a large dataset containing naturally occurring medical conversations video-recorded in clinical settings (Stivers, 2005). After identifying these practices, their impact on antibiotic prescribing was investigated. The findings revealed that providing both negative and positive treatment recommendations (as opposed to one or none) is associated with a decrease in inappropriate antibiotic prescribing (Mangione-Smith et al., 2015).

Communication behavior 2: *Ending visits with a contingency plan.*

The *contingency plan* is a practice to recommend for what parents can do if their child's condition worsens or shows no improvement over the following 2–3 days. For example, "Definitely call me if she starts having high fevers. I don't expect that to happen, but that's what you should watch for."

The evaluation of the DART program showed that training clinicians to change their communication behaviors, including delivering a two-part treatment recommendation (negative plus positive) and offering a contingency plan, significantly reduced overall antibiotic prescribing and inappropriate prescribing for children with ARTIs in pediatric outpatient settings (Kronman et al., 2020; Mangione-Smith et al., 2015). Moreover, it is also found that clinicians' use of this communication strategy is positively associated with parents' increased visit satisfaction (Mangione-Smith et al., 2001, 2015).

These successful experiences demonstrate the importance of understanding doctor–patient interaction in clinical settings. They also show that equipping doctors with evidence-based communication techniques have great potential to reduce inappropriate antibiotic prescribing. Although these findings were made in the Western clinical context, having a deep understanding of doctor-caregiver interaction in prescribing decision-making and designing evidence-based intervention programs also have implications for reducing inappropriate antibiotic prescribing in Chinese pediatric primary care. In this regard, the studies presented in this book serve as a starting point.

Countering pressure in Chinese pediatrics: two communication opportunities

There are features unique to the Chinese settings that may require specific intervention measures. First, Chinese doctors have considerably less medical authority compared to Western settings. In China, patients/caregivers demonstrate a higher level of entitlement in advocating for antibiotics and initiating treatment negotiations with their doctors during medical encounters. This suggests that it is important to reshape the doctor–patient relationship and rebuild trust between doctors and patients in China.

Second, not only do patient caregivers demonstrate a higher level of entitlement to negotiate with their doctors during medical visits, but they also show a lack of understanding regarding the consequences of the misuse and overuse of antibiotics. Rather than considering antibiotics as prescription medicine with restricted use and access, they view them as a common commodity, similar to Mentos candy, that they can freely use and purchase at community pharmacy stores or order in the consultation room. This suggests that there is an ongoing need for educating patients and caregivers about the rational use of antibiotics.

In fact, public health education campaigns promoting the rational use of antibiotics have been implemented for years. However, their effects have been found to be limited. Findings of this book demonstrate that when caregivers bring their children to visit doctors, they still demand antibiotics and IV treatment. This does not mean that educational campaigns among patients and caregivers are without value. Instead, it highlights the urgent need to explore additional methods to educate patients and caregivers about the importance of rational antibiotic use.

The doctor–patient interaction offers an important opportunity to shape patients' and caregivers' understanding of illness and conduct educational campaigns on the rational use of antibiotics. In the following, I will introduce two types of opportunities in medical interaction that are highly relevant to the Chinese pediatric primary care setting.

Opportunity 1: *Online commentary: Foreshadowing viral diagnosis and non-antibiotic treatment in physical examinations.*

Online commentary is a communication behavior that is widely used in American pediatric outpatient settings. It is identified as a potential strategy to reduce patient resistance to treatment recommendation and inappropriate antibiotic prescription (Heritage et al., 2010; Mangione-Smith et al., 2003). This communication behavior mainly involves the doctor describing what he or she is finding during the physical examination of the patient.

Studies have found that doctors use this communication behavior to forecast the likely results of the physical examination during the examination itself (Heritage & Stivers, 1999). In the context of pediatric outpatient care, it can be used to forecast a bacterial or viral diagnosis and, consequently, foreshadow a potential antibiotic or non-antibiotic treatment for the patient.

Specifically, two primary types of *online commentaries* were observed. First, *'problem' online commentary* is suggestive of a problematic finding on physical examination that might require antibiotic treatment. For example, the doctor might say, "That cough sounds very chesty." Second, *'no-problem' online commentary* indicates physical examination findings that were not problematic and that antibiotics were probably not necessary. For instance, the doctor might say, "Her throat is only slightly red."

Building on this conversation analysis research, scholars have conducted further investigations into the relationship between the communication behavior of online commentary and inappropriate antibiotic prescribing. Overall, the findings showed that the communication behavior of online commentary during the physical examination was widely used in clinical interaction, occurring in 71% of visits with viral diagnoses.

In addition, the scholars found that doctors' use of *'problem'* and *'no-problem' online commentaries* had differential impacts on antibiotic prescribing outcomes. For presumed viral cases where the doctor thought the parent expected to receive antibiotics, if the doctor used at least some *'problem' online commentary*, s/he prescribed antibiotics in 91% of cases. Conversely, when the doctor exclusively employed *'no problem' online commentary*, antibiotics were prescribed 27% of the time. Compared to similar cases with *'no problem' online commentary*, *'problem' online commentary* was associated with a 27% greater probability of an inappropriate antibiotic prescription.

Moreover, the series of studies also showed that doctors' use of *'no problem' online commentary* did not significantly increase the length of the visit. This suggests that *'no problem' online commentary* is a communication technique that can be easily incorporated into doctors' routine communication practices to reduce inappropriate antibiotic prescribing.

Opportunity 2: *Responding to resistance: Creating teachable moments for rational antibiotic use following caregiver resistance.*

Given the high frequency of patient caregivers resisting doctors' treatment recommendations in the Chinese pediatric settings and the significant impact this has on antibiotic inappropriate prescribing, it is important to consider how to effectively respond to caregiver resistance.

To date, no research has been conducted to investigate the effect of any particular type of doctor's response to caregiver resistance in reducing inappropriate antibiotic prescribing. However, a conversation analysis study examining the sequential unfolding of talk following patient resistance suggests that effective responses from doctors not only have the potential to reduce inappropriate antibiotic prescribing but also to build supportive relationships between doctors and patient caregivers.

Rather than treating a patient caregiver's resistance as a negative interactional event where conflicting stances are taken regarding the patient's treatment plan, challenging the doctor's medical authority, doctors can consider it as an important opportunity (Wang, 2023). This opportunity allows them to (1) understand the perspectives and challenges of patient and caregivers regarding the illness and treatment and (2) provide targeted education on rational use of antibiotics to patients and caregivers.

*(1) Caregiver resistance: an opportunity to learn about patient caregiver's
perspective and challenges*

Excerpt 7.1 illustrates a case in point. In this excerpt, the patient complains about mild coughing over the past two days. The doctor diagnoses the condition as a cold with some signs of bronchitis and recommends an oral medication treatment (lines 1–2). Following the recommendation, the caregiver withholds her acceptance by remaining silent for a noticeable period (line 3). Subsequently, the mother switches to overtly resisting the doctor's oral treatment recommendation by nominating an alternative treatment for the patient (line 4).

Excerpt 7.1 An example of resistance displaying a caregiver's perspective on the treatment

D: Doctor
M: Mother

1	D:	感冒,	有点	气管	炎症.	
		ganmao	youdian	qiguan	yanzheng	
		cold	a little	airway	inflammation	
		"(He's got) a cold,				
2		吃	点	药	吧?	
		chi	dian	yao	ba	
		take	some	medication	PT	
		a little inflammation in the airway."				
3->		(4.0)				
4=>	**M:**	不	挂水	啊?		
		bu	guashui	a		
		no	drip	PT		
		"No drip?"				
5	D:	呃,	挂水	不	需要	吧,
		e	guashui	bu	xuyao	ba
		uh	drip	no	need	PT
		"Uh, drip, no need for drip."				

Through passive resistance (line 3), the mother does not align herself with the doctor's proposed plan of treatment, indicating a preference against the non-antibiotic treatment. Through active resistance (line 4), the mother not only disaffiliates with the doctor on the treatment plan but also demonstrates her understanding of the patient's condition and her own opinion on the proper course of treatment. The proposed antibiotic IV treatment is at least relevant to the patient's condition, if not better suited or preferred compared to the recommended oral treatment.

In addition to providing valuable information on caregivers' perspective and treatment preferences, caregivers' resistance also allows for the disclosure of information about the life circumstances of the patients and the caregivers.

In Excerpt 7.2, the patient visits the doctor due to a cough that has persisted for over two weeks. The patient also experiences sneezing and nasal congestion symptoms. After reviewing the X-ray and blood tests results, the doctor does not find any clear signs of *Mycoplasma pneumoniae* – a severe infection condition that requires antibiotic treatment. As a result, she suggests starting the patient on oral antibiotic treatment (lines 2–4). However, this treatment recommendation is resisted by both the mother (lines 5–7) and the grandmother (lines 9–10, lines 12–14), expressing concern about the child's difficulty in taking oral medicine.

Excerpt 7.2 Active resistance: difficulty in taking medicine

1		((A few lines of blood test results discussion omitted))					
2	D:	你	就算	要是	没	口服	过	药,
		ni	Jiusuan	yaoshi	mei	koufu	guo	yao
		you	even	if	not	oral	that	medicine
		"Even if you haven't taken any oral medicine yet,						
3		你	给	他	吃	点	那个	阿奇霉素
		ni	gei	ta	chi	dian	nage	aqimeisu
		you	give	him	take	some	that	*Azithromycin*
		you can give him some oral azithromycin take.						
4		也	行,	口服.				
		ye	xing	koufu				
		also	fine	oral				
		It would also do. Oral medication."						
5->	**M:**	我	家里	吧,	口服	药	全	有,
		wo	jiali	ba	koufu	yao	quan	you
		My	home	PRT	oral	medicine	all	have
		"I have all those oral medicine at home.						
6->		[然后	他	不	吃:,			
		ranhou	Ta	bu	chi			
		then	He	not	take			
		and he doesn't take it.						
7->		一	吃	完	就	吐.		
		yi	chi	wan	jiu	tu		
		once	take	up	then	vomit		
		He'll vomit once he finishes taking the oral medicine."						
8	D:	[但	他	吃	不	进去,		
		dan	Ta	chi	bu	jinqu		

Excerpt 7.2 (Continued)

		but	He	take	not	in			
		"But he can't take it in."							
9->	**GM:**	他	一	吃	完	就	吐,		
		ta	Yi	chi	wan	jiu	tu		
		he	once	take	up	then	vomit		
		"He'll vomit once he finishes taking the oral medicine.							
10->		哎呀,	吐	那	到处	都	是.		
		aiya	Tu	na	daochu	dou	shi		
		alas	vomit	there	everywhere	all	is		
		Alas. He vomited everywhere."							
11	D:	那	你	吐	完	再	喂	呢?	
		na	Ni	tu	wan	zai	wei	ne	
		then	you	vomit	over	again	feed	PRT	
		"Then what about you feed him again after he finishes vomiting?"							
12->	**GM:**	再	喂	也	不	行,			
		zai	wei	ye	bu	xing			
		again	feed	also	not	alright			
		"Feeding him again won't work.							
13->		不	吃	了	那	就,	也	不	吃,
		bu	chi	le	na	jiu	ye	bu	chi
		not	take	PRT	that	then	also	not	take
		He won't take it then, won't take it again.							
14->		我	喂	也	喂	不	进去.		
		wo	wei	ye	wei	bu	jinqu		
		I	feed	also	feed	not	in		
		I can't feed it in, even if I feed him again."							
15	D:	那	你	就	输	点	滴流,	要不-	
		na	Ni	jiu	shu	dian	diliu	yaobu	
		then	you	then	give	some	drip	otherwise	
		"Then you just have some IV drip, otherwise."							
16	M:	打	两	天	滴流	呗.			
		da	liang	tian	diliu	bei			
		have	two	day	drip	PRT			
		"Have two-days' drip."							

The concern, which arises from the caregiver's real-world experiences, does not take issue with the doctor's clinical judgment of the patient's condition or the effectiveness of the suggested treatment. In line 11, the doctor pursues the caregivers' (mother and grandmother) acceptance by suggesting that the patient's obstacle can be overcome through feeding attempts. Although the doctor's fails to gain acceptance from the caregivers (line 14), this case highlights the valuable opportunity that patient resistance affords for the doctor to learn about the patient's opinions and obstacles related to their illness and treatment.

(2) Response to resistance: an opportunity to conduct targeting patient/caregiver education on rational use of antibiotics

Patient resistance not only provides valuable insights into patients' perspectives and life circumstances but also offers doctors significant opportunities to discuss rational antibiotic use with them.

Excerpt 7.3 provides an example of the caregiver's resistance, which is then followed by the doctor providing knowledge about the rational use of IV antibiotic treatment. The excerpt is the same with Excerpt 7.2. As mentioned earlier, the doctor's treatment recommendation of oral medication is initially met with passive, then active resistance (line 4). While the caregiver's passive resistance indicates hesitation toward the treatment recommendation, it does not reveal the grounds for the resistance. In contrast, active resistance reveals the caregiver's perspective on what she believes is relevant or preferred for treating the patient's condition. Following this, the doctor pursues the caregiver's acceptance by addressing the caregiver's perspective and preference. Specifically, the doctor first denies the need for the IV treatment (line 5) and provides a rationale for her recommended treatment (line 6–7).

Excerpt 7.3 An example of active resistance followed by doctor's provision of a rationale

M: Mother
D: Doctor

4	M:	不	挂水	啊?				
		bu	guashui	a				
		no	Drip	PT				
		"No drip?"						
5->	**D:**	呃,	挂水	不	需要	吧,		
		e	guashui	bu	xuyao	ba		
		uh	Drip	no	need	PT		
		"Uh, no need for drip.						
6->		先	吃	点	药.	能	吃	药	好
		xian	Chi	dian	yao	neng	chi	yao	hao
		first	Take	some	medication	can	take	medication	well
		Take some (oral) medication first. (If he) can get well with oral medication,							
7->		就	尽量	吃	药	好.			
		jiu	jinliang	chi	yao	hao			
		then	Best	take	medication	well			
		just try the best to take oral medication, OK?"							
8	M:	哦,	好.						
		o	Hao						
		okay	OK						
		"OK, OK."							

Note that, on the one hand, the doctor's response (lines 5–7) serves to counter the parental pressure for IV treatment. On the other hand, it helps the caregiver understand the reasoning behind the doctor's treatment recommendation and the standard approach for managing similar conditions. Upon receiving this new information, the mother accepts the doctor's original recommendation for oral treatment (line 8). This demonstrates that while caregiver resistance presents a significant challenge to the doctor (in this case, it even puts the progressivity of the consultation on halt), it also presents a valuable opportunity for doctors to educate caregivers about the rational use of medicine and for caregivers to become more informed about treatment decisions.

Excerpt 7.4 provides an example of a doctor's response to a caregiver's passive resistance, providing additional information about the patient's condition and the recommended treatment. In this example, the child visits the doctor due to a fever. Prior to the visit, the caregivers had already administered oral medication to the child. Upon finding no signs of bacterial infection, the doctor suggests the patient continue using the same oral medication as before the visit (lines 1–2). However, this recommendation is met with passive resistance from the caregivers at line 3. In response, the doctor pursues the caregivers' acceptance by discussing the patient's blood test result (lines 4–6).

Excerpt 7.4 An example of doctor's response to caregiver passive resistance

D: Doctor
GM1: Grandmother (both grandmothers are present, GM1 refers to the first one to speak)

1	D:	实际上	啊,	你	这个			
		Shijishang	a	ni	zhege			
		Actually	PT	you	this			
		"Actually, with this (blood test result),						
2		还	要	继续	吃	药.		
		hai	yao	jixu	chi	yao		
		still	need	continue	take	medication		
		you still need to go on taking (oral) medication."						
3		(.)						
4=>	**D:**	[你	这个	血象	啊-			
		ni	zhege	xuexiang	a			
		you	this	hemogram	PT			
		"Your hemogram-"						
5	GM1:	[没的	用	哎,				
		meide	yong	ai				
		no	use	PT				
		"It won't work."						
6=>	**D:**	你	这个	血象	也	不	高	哎,
		ni	zhege	xuexiang	ye	bu	gao	ai
		you	this	hemogram	also	not	high	PT
		"Your hemogram (value) isn't high."						

The doctor's pursuit of the caregivers' acceptance involves first referring to the test result (line 4) and then providing the rationale for the recommended treatment, emphasizing the non-problematic nature of the test result (line 6). By providing additional information about the patient's condition and the diagnostic test, the doctor shares information that is important for the caregivers' understanding of the child's condition and the rationale behind the recommended treatment.

Excerpt 7.5 further demonstrates how a doctor's response to a caregiver's resistance can assist patients and caregivers in comprehending the nature of the condition and the characteristics of medication. In this excerpt, the doctor's pursuit of the caregiver's acceptance (line 6) is once again met with resistance from the caregiver (line 7). This resistance an other-initiated repair (Drew, 1997), with the caregiver partly repeating the doctor's previous statement, putting the flow of the conversation on halt. To address this resistance, the doctor proceeds to discuss the specific value of the blood test, offering an explanation for her diagnosis and the recommended treatment (line 8).

Excerpt 7.5 An example of doctor's response to caregiver active resistance

D: Doctor

GM2: Grandmother (both grandmothers are present, GM2 refers to the second one to speak)

6	D:	你	这个	血象		也	不	高	哎,
		Ni	zhege	xuexiang		ye	bu	gao	ai
		You	this	hemogram		also	not	high	PT
		"Your hemogram (value) isn't high."							
7->	GM2:	不	高	是	啊?=				
		bu	gao	shi	a				
		not	high	is	PRT				
		"Not high, is it?"							
8=>	**D:**	嗯,	才	五千	多.				
		En	cai	wuqian	duo				
		yeah	only	five-thousand	over				
		"Yeah, it's just over five-thousand."							
9->	GM1:	哎,	对的	哎,					
		ai	duide	ai					
		yeah	right	PRT					
		"Yeah, right."							
10->		我家	吃	药	吃	不	住	哎.	
		Wojia	chi	yao	chi	bu	zhu	ai	
		ours	take	medicine	take	not	down	PRT	
		"Oral medicine can't bring it down for us."							
11->	GM2:	挂	两	天	水-				
		gua	liang	tian	shui				
		drip	two	day	drip				
		"Have two-days' drip."							
12=>	**D:**	你	挂	两	天	水,			
		ni	gua	liang	tian	shui			
		you	drip	two	day	drip			
		"You have two-days' drip.							
13=>		挂	那个-	抗病毒的,					
		gua	nage-	kangbingdude					

(*Continued*)

Excerpt 7.5 (Continued)

		drip	that	anti-viral				
		Use that anti-viral medicine for drip.						
14=>		你	挂	那个	头孢	实际上	也	没用.
		Ni	gua	nage	toubao	shijishang	ye	meiyong
		you	drip	that	Cephlo	actually	also	useless
		(If) you use Cephalo for drip, it doesn't really help."						

Although the caregiver (GM1) acknowledges the doctor's professional judgment (line 9), she resists by asserting that the patient's specific circumstance may differ from the general situation (line 10). This active resistance is further supported by the other caregiver (GM2), with an explicit request for an alternative treatment, *Have two-days drip* (line 11). In response to the caregivers' active resistance, the doctor negatively assesses the requested treatment (IV antibiotics/Cephalo) by stating, *If you use Cephalo for drip, it doesn't really help* (lines 12–14). The doctor, thus, denies the need for the IV treatment and further pursues the caregivers' acceptance of the initial treatment recommendation. As shown in this example, the caregivers' resistance prompts the doctor to provide further information about the patient's condition and the recommended treatment.

Excerpt 7.6 provides another example of a caregiver's resistance, prompting the doctor to provide more information about the rational use of antibiotics for the caregiver's self-management of the patient's common condition in her everyday life. Given the high prevalence of non-prescribed antibiotic use in the community, this information is crucial for reducing the misuse and overuse of antibiotics outside of clinical settings.

In this example, the patient is brought in for a cough and sore throat. Before the doctor's visit, the caregiver has already given the child Dalifen (*cefixime*), an oral antibiotic. However, since the physical examination does not show signs of a bacterial infection, the doctor recommends oral treatment for the patient (line 1). The mother actively resists this recommendation with a partial repeat (line 2), to which the doctor responds with a provision of information regarding the timing of antibiotic use (line 3–4).

Excerpt 7.6 An example of caregiver's display of perspective through active resistance

D: Doctor
M: Mother

1	D:	你:,	吃	点	药	吧.
		ni	chi	dian	yao	ba
		you	take	some	medicine	PRT
		"You, how about you take some oral medicine?"				

Excerpt 7.6 (Continued)

2->	M:	吃	点	药	啊?		
		chi	dian	yao	a		
		take	some	medicine	PRT		
		"Take some oral medicine?"					

3=>	**D:**	哎,	你	前面	达力芬	其实	刚	开始
		ai	ni	qianmian	Dalifen	qishi	gang	kaishi
		yeah	you	before	Dalifen	actually	just	beginning

4=>		倒	不	要	吃.
		dao	bu	yao	chi
		contrary	not	need	take
		"Yeah, actually you don't have to take Dalifen before,			
		at the very beginning."			

In the face of the mother's active resistance, the doctor first confirms the treatment recommendation with *ai* ("yeah"). She then criticizes the caregiver's decision to self-medicate the patient with oral antibiotics before the visit, emphasizing that antibiotics or IV treatment are not necessary. Therefore, when the caregiver resists, doctors not only have opportunity to address the caregiver's indicated treatment preferences but also to share important knowledge about the rational use of antibiotics and management of the patient's common conditions.

In sum, while it is widely acknowledged that resistance from patients is an important resource when promoting shared decision-making (SDM), patient or caregiver resistance is often viewed as a negative event in practice. Rather than avoiding or preempting it, the prior examples suggest that resistance can also present a valuable opportunity for doctors and patient caregivers to foster shared understanding, establish a supportive relationship, and reduce the inappropriate use of antibiotics both within and outside the clinical setting. A minor shift in the mindset is likely to do the magic.

Concluding remarks

In her World Health Day 2011 speech, WHO Director-General Chan also mentioned, "We have taken antibiotics for granted. And we have failed to handle these fragile medicines with appropriate care." This is what this book aims to demonstrate and explain – the social and interactional nature of antibiotic overprescription. The following three core messages are summarized as the conclusion of this book.

First, antibiotic prescribing decisions, what may seem like a purely biomedical decision, are affected by the interaction between doctors and patient caregivers in medical encounters. The decision to prescribe antibiotics is made in and through doctor-caregiver interaction rather than being predetermined by factors such as doctors' incentives to profit from overprescribing. The outcome of prescribing decisions is not solely determined by the doctors but is significantly influenced by perceived or actual pressure from caregivers conveyed in medical interaction.

Second, antibiotic prescribing decisions, what may seem like a purely professional decision, are affected by a complex matrix of social factors. At the micro-level, prescribing decisions are often influenced by patients' or caregivers' behaviors, attitudes, and personal preferences. At the macro-level, these behaviors, attitudes, and preferences are also influenced by historical and institutional arrangements of the healthcare system as well as the resulting medical culture.

Third, antibiotic overprescription, a problem that stems from social and interactional factors, can also be resolved by addressing these factors. By training and applying essential communication skills in clinical practices, doctors can effectively handle the interactional pressure from patient caregivers for inappropriate antibiotic prescriptions. Through understanding the pivotal moments in medical decision-making and creating teachable moments in medical interaction, doctors have opportunities to shape patients' and caregivers' understanding of their illness and raise awareness of the rational use of medicine.

References

Cabral, C., Horwood, J., Symonds, J., Ingram, J., Lucas, P. J., Redmond, N. M., Kai, J., Hay, A. D., & Barnes, R. K. (2019). Understanding the influence of parent-clinician communication on antibiotic prescribing for children with respiratory tract infections in primary care: A qualitative observational study using a conversation analysis approach. *BMC Family Practice, 20*(1), 102. https://doi.org/10.1186/s12875-019-0993-9

Dialogue Around Respiratory Illness Treatment (DART). (2016). https://www.uwimtr.org/dart/

Drew, P. (1997). 'Open' class repair initiators in response to sequential sources of troubles in conversation. *Journal of Pragmatics, 28*(1), 69–101. https://doi.org/10.1016/S0378-2166(97)89759-7

Heritage, J., Elliott, M. N., Stivers, T., Richardson, A., & Mangione-Smith, R. (2010). Reducing inappropriate antibiotics prescribing: The role of online commentary on physical examination findings. *Patient Education and Counseling, 81*(1), 119–125.

Heritage, J., & Stivers, T. (1999). Online commentary in acute medical visits: A method of shaping patient expectations. *Social Science & Medicine (1982), 49*(11), 1501–1517.

Kronman, M. P., Gerber, J. S., Grundmeier, R. W., Zhou, C., Robinson, J. D., Heritage, J., Stout, J., Burges, D., Hedrick, B., Warren, L., Shalowitz, M., Shone, L. P., Steffes, J., Wright, M., Fiks, A. G., & Mangione-Smith, R. (2020). Reducing antibiotic prescribing in primary care for respiratory illness. *Pediatrics, 146*(3). https://doi.org/10.1542/peds.2020-0038

Mangione-Smith, R., McGlynn, E., Elliott, N., McDonald, L., Franz, L., & Kravitz, L. (2001). Parent expectations for antibiotics, physician-parent communication, and satisfaction. *Archives of Pediatrics and Adolescent Medicine, 155*(7), 800–806.

Mangione-Smith, R., Robinson, J. D., Zhou, C., Stout, J. W., Fiks, A. G., Shalowitz, M., Gerber, J. S., Burges, D., Hedrick, B., Warren, L., Grundmeier, R. W., Kronman, M. P., Shone, L. P., Steffes, J., Wright, M., & Heritage, J. (2022). Fidelity evaluation of the dialogue around respiratory illness treatment (DART) program communication training. *Patient Education and Counseling, 105*(7), 2611–2616. https://doi.org/10.1016/j.pec.2022.03.011

Mangione-Smith, R., Stivers, T., Elliott, N., McDonald, L., & Heritage, J. (2003). Online commentary during the physical examination: A communication tool for avoiding inappropriate antibiotic prescribing? *Social Science & Medicine*, *56*(2), 313–320.

Mangione-Smith, R., Zhou, C., Robinson, J. D., Taylor, J. A., Elliott, M. N., & Heritage, J. (2015). Communication practices and antibiotic use for acute respiratory tract infections in children. *Annals of Family Medicine*, *13*(3), 221–227. https://doi.org/10.1370/afm.1785

Parsons, T. (1951). *Social system*. Routledge.

Stivers, T. (2005). Non-antibiotic treatment recommendations: Delivery formats and implications for parent resistance. *Social Science & Medicine*, *5*(60), 949–964.

Stivers, T., Mangione-Smith, R., Elliott, M. N., McDonald, L., & Heritage, J. (2003). Why do physicians think parents expect antibiotics? What parents report vs what physicians believe. *The Journal of Family Practice*, *52*(2), 140–147.

Wang, N. C. (2023). Resistance to treatment recommendations: An interactional resource to increase information exchange and promote shared decision-making in medical encounters. In *Language, health and culture*. Routledge.

Appendix

Notes on medical interaction data and conversation analysis

Naturally occurring medical interaction data

Pediatrics is where antibiotics are most frequently prescribed and overprescription is most likely to happen (Hales et al., 2018; Hui et al., 1997; Vernacchio et al., 2009; Wang et al., 2020). Between October and December 2013, 318 video-recorded pediatric encounters for children's respiratory tract infection conditions were collected. The dataset involves 318 patients with their caregivers, 9 doctors (8 female, 1 male), and 6 hospitals at 3 tiers in urban areas in China. Among them, 196 are acute visits, in which the patient has not been seen previously by the doctor for the primary condition under consultation. Each conversation is 4.9 minutes on average, and the total length of the recordings is 26 hours.

For the purpose of comparing my findings to studies conducted in similar settings, I used a subset of the 196 video recordings containing medical encounters for acute visits only. Among them, 9 visits were excluded from analysis because of incompleteness or inaudible utterances in the target turns at talk. This results in 187 acute pediatric visits for analysis. Although both patients and caregivers are present in the medical encounters, the conversations are mostly between doctors and caregivers. Children's contribution is very limited.

Data are transcribed following conversation analytic (CA) conventions (Jefferson, 2004), mainly capturing paralinguistic features of the turn, such as intonation, over-laps, and cut-offs. Four-line formatted transcripts are provided in the paper, including the Chinese verbatim, Pinyin, word-for-word translation, and gloss translation. Each conversation is analyzed at the turn level, determining whether its primary social action is a treatment recommendation or a response to a treatment recommendation.

This results in a corpus of transcribed medical conversations of 468,162 Chinese characters and 39,216 turns in total. Detailed analytical procedures relating to caregiver advocating practices for antibiotic prescriptions, doctors' treatment recommendation actions, and treatment recommendation-response sequences in medical interaction are presented separately in Chapter 4, Chapter 5, and Chapter 6.

The University of California, Los Angeles (UCLA) Institutional Review Board (IRB) approved all procedures for the duration of the study (IRB#13-000748). No identifiable information was involved in the study.

Conversation analysis

In Chapter 4, Chapter 5, and Chapter 6, conversation analysis (CA) is used as the primary methodology to identify caregivers' and doctors' interactional behaviors in naturally occurring conversations. Here, I provide a brief introduction of the method to explain (1) how CA can be used to analyze participants' actions in social encounters, (2) how CA can be used to analyze the social relationship between the actors who produce these actions, and (3) how CA can be used in combination with quantitative analysis for building arguments.

CA as a method to analyze social actions

Inspired by Erving Goffman and Harold Garfinkel, CA was developed in 1960s by Harvey Sacks, Emanuel Schegloff, and colleagues as a rigorous approach to the study of social interactions and, more essentially, social orders. At its core, CA assumes that there may be order at all points in social activities (Sacks et al., 1974). For conversation analysts, conversation is just one form of social activity which is directly accessible and the very details of actual social events and conducts could be captured in their entirety and re-examined repeatedly (Drew et al., 2001). Thus, researchers taking a CA approach rely on video/audio recordings of naturally occurring conversations and detailed transcripts of them.

An extensive body of theory and empirical research has been devoted to showing that there is normative structuring and shared logics underlying participants' courses of actions in conversation and that such a 'micro-order' of social interactions not only makes possible the intelligibility of the social actions (Heritage, 2005) but also forms the very foundations of the so-called 'macro-order' of society (Schegloff, 2006). It is in this sense that CA was developed as a method to serve the broader enterprise of building a stable, reproducible, cumulative, natural observational science of social action and, hence, of society (Drew et al., 2001; Sacks, 1985; Schegloff, 1987).

Specifically, the 'micro-order' or structural organization of conversation can be operationalized at three different levels in conversation: First, actions: the main job being undertaken in a turn. Rather than being primarily concerned with what words and other language particulars 'mean,' conversation analysis focuses on the function that turns have including what sort of response is invited or even normatively required by a given action. Next, sequences: how a sequence of turns is organized in a trajectory, through which courses of action are enacted coherently and orderly. For example, "Are you free tonight?" can be understood as a preliminary to a base adjacency pair of invitation-acceptance. Sequences are the vehicle for getting activities accomplished (Schegloff, 2007; Stivers, 2010). Finally, overall organization: how multiple, ordered sequences are organized to accomplish a particular project (e.g., a medical project normally involves six ordered activities – problem presentation, history-taking, physical examination, diagnosis, treatment, closing) (Robinson, 2012; Schegloff, 2007).

In addition to this structural view of conversation, there is also a dimension of morality in the systematic organization of social interactions. Related work encompasses preference organization (Pomerantz, 1984; Pomerantz & Heritage, 2012), repair organization (Kitzinger, 2012; Schegloff et al., 1977), and displays and negotiations of epistemic authority (Heritage & Raymond, 2005, 2012) and deontic authority (Stevanovic & Peräkylä, 2012).

The systematic organization of conversation is fundamental to the smooth functioning of society, as participants constantly rely on conversation's organizational resources as shared sensemaking practices in producing and understanding actions with each other (Maynard & Heritage, 2023). What is intriguing about this sensemaking process is that whether an action of a speaker is understood as performing a particular action is not only discernable to the participants in the listener's subsequent turn but is also discernable to the analysts simultaneously – an analytical procedure called 'a next turn proof procedure' in CA. For this reason, CA is used as the primary methodology to identify the actions and the sequences that doctors and patient caregivers use and rely on to make prescribing decisions in medical encounters.

CA as a method to analyze social relationships

Related to this sensemaking process that involves the participants' shared knowledge and practices of systematic organization of conversation is their reliance on the analyses of the contextual knowledge of the social relationship, the local interactional environment, and the larger activity in which the participants are engaged (Pomerantz & Mandelbaum, 2004). Particularly, as Pomerantz and Mandelbaum (2004) put it: "Persons assume that incumbents of specific relationship categories should conduct themselves in ways that are consistent with the rights, obligations, motives, and activities regarded as proper for incumbents of the relationship categories or be accountable for the discrepancy" (p.150).

Since its inception, CA has investigated how participants put their knowledge of relationship categories to use in interaction and how the knowledge, understanding, and assumptions related to relationship categories are drawn on in the normal course of accountable social and work-related activities. Although enacting incumbency in a relationship category is not the focal activity in most cases, sensitivity to incumbency in a relationship may account for the particular ways in which these actions are implemented (Pomerantz & Mandelbaum, 2004, p. 167). Thus, by looking at the ways that actions are implemented, we can also understand the kind of social relationship at play and the kind of incumbents associated with the relationship categories. In this study, CA is used to examine not only the interactional processes and actions through which antibiotic prescribing decisions are made but also the social relationship between doctors and patient caregivers, which underlies their interactional behaviors and indirectly contributes to the overprescription problem.

Combining conversation analysis and quantitative analysis

Based on the conversation analysis of medical interaction dataset, I also conduct quantitative analysis to examine the bivariate relationships between the conversation actions and variables such as prescribing outcomes. In particular, I use CA as a basis for operationalizing variables that can then be coded. Once coded, I am able to test for associations between the actions that are identified and the outcome variables that are of interest. This mixed methodology thus aims to provide not only a qualitative understanding of the interactional actions or processes that are identified as influencing the antibiotic overprescription problem but also a quantitative estimation of the significance of the associations between the actions and the prescribing outcomes.

Table A.1 Transcription symbols for conversation analysis

Symbol	Features of talk represented
(.)	A dot in a parentheses indicates a pause of less than two-tenths of a second
(0.5)	Numbers in parentheses refer to pauses in tenths of a second
:	Colons indicate an extension of the preceding vowel sound; the more colons, the greater the extent of the stretching
[	Square brackets indicate the beginning of overlapping talk
–	A dash following a word indicates a cut-off of talk
=	Equal signs indicate continuous talk between speakers
.	Final falling intonation
,	Slight rising intonation
?	Sharp rising intonation
((description))	Double parentheses contain descriptions of physical movement or non-verbal activity

References

Drew, P., Chatwin, J., & Collins, S. (2001). Conversation analysis: A method for research into interactions between patients and health-care professionals. *Health Expectations: An International Journal of Public Participation in Health Care and Health Policy*, *4*(1), 58–70. https://doi.org/10.1046/j.1369-6513.2001.00125.x

Hales, C. M., Kit, B. K., Gu, Q., & Ogden, C. L. (2018). Trends in prescription medication use among children and adolescents – United States, 1999–2014. *JAMA*, *319*(19), 2009–2020. https://doi.org/10.1001/jama.2018.5690

Heritage, J., & Raymond, G. (2005). The terms of agreement: Indexing epistemic authority and subordination in talk-in-interaction. *Social Psychology Quarterly*, *68*(1), 15–38. https://doi.org/10.1177/019027250506800103

Heritage, J., & Raymond, G. (2012). Navigating epistemic landscapes: Acquiescence, agency and resistance in responses to polar questions. In *Questions: Formal, functional and interactional perspectives* (pp. 179–192). Cambridge University Press.

Hui, L., Li, X. S., Zeng, X., Dai, Y., & Foy, H. (1997). Patterns and determinants of use of antibiotics for acute respiratory tract infection in children in China. *The Pediatric Infectious Disease Journal*, *16*(6), 560–564.

Jefferson, G. (2004). Glossary of transcript symbols with an introduction. In *Conversation analysis: Studies from the first generation* (pp. 13–31). John Benjamins.

Kitzinger, C. (2012). Repair. In *The handbook of conversation analysis* (pp. 229–256). Wiley-Blackwell.

Mandelbaum, A. P., Jenny. (2004). Conversation Analytic Approaches to the Relevance and Uses of Relationship Categories in Interaction. In Kristine L. Fitch & Robert E. Sanders (Eds.), *Handbook of Language and Social Interaction*. Psychology Press.

Maynard, D. W., & Heritage, J. (2023). Ethnomethodology's legacies and prospects. *Annual Review of Sociology*, *49*(1), 59–80. https://doi.org/10.1146/annurev-soc-020321-033738

Pomerantz, A. (1984). *Agreeing and disagreeing with assessments: Some features of preferred/dispreferred turn shaped*. Communication Faculty Scholarship. http://scholarsarchive.library.albany.edu/cas_communication_scholar/3

Pomerantz, A., & Heritage, J. (2012). Preference. In *The handbook of conversation analysis* (pp. 210–228). Wiley-Blackwell.

Robinson, J. D. (2012). Overall structural organization. In J. Sidnell & T. Stivers (Eds.), *The handbook of conversation analysis* (pp. 257–280). John Wiley & Sons, Ltd. https://doi.org/10.1002/9781118325001.ch13

Sacks, H. (1985). Notes on methodology. In J. M. Atkinson (Ed.), *Structures of social action* (pp. 21–27). Cambridge University Press. https://doi.org/10.1017/CBO9780511665868.005

Sacks, H., Schegloff, E., & Jefferson, G. (1974). A simplest systematics for the organization of turn-taking for conversation. *Language*, *50*, 696–735.

Schegloff, E. A. (1987). Analyzing single episodes of interaction: An exercise in conversation analysis. *Social Psychology Quarterly*, *50*(2), 101–114. https://doi.org/10.2307/2786745

Schegloff, E. (2007). *Sequence organization in interaction: A primer in conversation analysis*. Cambridge University Press.

Schegloff, E. A. (2006). Interaction: The Infrastructure for Social Institutions, the Natural Ecological Niche for Language, and the Arena in which Culture is Enacted. In Stephen C. Levinson & Nicholas J. Enfield (Eds.), *Roots of Human Sociality*. Routledge.

Schegloff, E., Jefferson, G., & Sacks, H. (1977). The preference for self-correction in the organisation of repair in conversation. *Language*, *53*, 361–382.

Stevanovic, M., & Peräkylä, A. (2012). Deontic authority in interaction: The right to announce, propose, and decide. *Research on Language & Social Interaction*, *45*(3), 297–321. https://doi.org/10.1080/08351813.2012.699260

Stivers, T. (2010). Sequence organization. In *The handbook of conversation analysis* (pp. 191–209). Wiley-Blackwell.

Vernacchio, L., Kelly, J. P., Kaufman, D. W., & Mitchell, A. A. (2009). Medication use among children <12 years of age in the United States: Results from the Slone survey. *Pediatrics*, *124*(2), 446–454. https://doi.org/10.1542/peds.2008-2869

Wang, C., Huttner, B. D., Magrini, N., Cheng, Y., Tong, J., Li, S., Wan, C., Zhu, Q., Zhao, S., Zhuo, Z., Lin, D., Yi, B., Shan, Q., Long, M., Jia, C., Zhao, D., Sun, X., Liu, J., Zhou, Y., . . . Hu, H. (2020). Pediatric antibiotic prescribing in China according to the 2019 World Health Organization Access, Watch, and Reserve (AWaRe) antibiotic categories. *The Journal of Pediatrics*, *220*, 125–131.e5. https://doi.org/10.1016/j.jpeds.2020.01.044

Index

Note: Numbers in **bold** indicate a table or an excerpt.

For Product Safety Concerns and Information please contact our EU
representative GPSR@taylorandfrancis.com
Taylor & Francis Verlag GmbH, Kaufingerstraße 24, 80331 München, Germany